17-DAY
GREEN TEA
DIET

Published in the United States by Galvanized Books, a division of Galvanized Brands, LLC, New York

Galvanized Books is a trademark of Galvanized Brands, LLC

ISBN 978-1-940358-06-2

Design by Mike Smith

Tea images by Shutterstock; Workout images by Beth Bischoff

GALVANIZED

17-DAY GREEN TEA DIET

TABLE OF CONTENTS

THE 17-DAY GREEN TEA DIET

FOREWORD

It seems incredible, Impossible...

And yet it's true: Fast, permanent weight loss is just a sip away. And all you need is a cup of hot water and a humble bag of green tea.

As the creator of Eat This, Not That!, the Editorial Director of *Shape* and *Men's Fitness* magazines, and the author of nearly two dozen best-selling books on nutrition, I've spent more than 20 years poring over fat-reduction programs, exercise plans, nutritional studies and every bit of body science that hits the journals. When it comes to weight-loss claims, you could call me the ultimate skeptic—but of course I'd ask for proof.

And as a skeptic, I can tell you this: Never before have I seen such a mountain of evidence that proves the effectiveness of a weight-loss plan. And never before have I found something so fast-acting, so foolproof, and so downright unassailably healthy for you. The *17-Day Green Tea Diet* will not only strip away fat—up to 14 pounds, from your belly first!—but it will put you on the path to a longer, healthier, richer life.

tea—in particular, a class of nutrients

cult to find in any other food source. This 17-day program unlocks those powerful nutrients by combining them with five very special superfoods, making them even more effective. As a result, this plan ushers you into an exclusive club—a club where everyone gets to lose weight and feel healthier, without restrictive dieting and without intensive exercise. And as they say, membership has its privileges:

> → **You live longer.** Those who drink the most green tea are less likely to die of any cause than those who do not, according to an 11-year study.

> → **You live leaner.** Green tea drinkers have, on average, 20 percent less body fat than non-drinkers.

> → **You live happier.** Green tea quashes hunger, lowers blood pressure, reduces stress and improves sleep, all while helping to cut your risk of the major disease of our time.

The *17-Day Green Tea Diet* is easy, it's incredibly inexpensive, and it works for everyone. Welcome to the club!

Now if you'll excuse me, I hear a teapot whistling....

—David Zinczenko
Creator and Founder, *Eat This, Not That!*

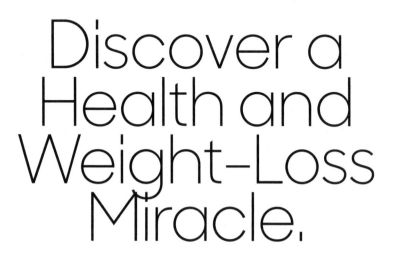

Discover a Health and Weight-Loss Miracle.

There's a weight-loss revolution brewing. And you are on the front lines!

You're about to learn the secret of the most effective weight-loss tool in the world—a weapon that works for everyone, costs just pennies a day, is available at any grocery store, requires no sweat or stress, and can be used at home, at work, or anywhere it's convenient.

That secret tool is green tea—a humble drink that's been cherished as a health miracle for centuries, but one that science is finally

Literally hundreds of studies have been carried out to document the health benefits of catechins, the group of antioxidants concentrated in the leaves of tea plants. And the most powerful of all catechins, a compound called epigallocatechin gallate, or EGCG, is found almost exclusively in green tea.

"I LOVED THE RESULTS! I FOLLOWED THE PLAN AND IN JUST SEVEN DAYS I LOST 9 POUNDS!"

—JEANNINE ARENAS, 31, MIAMI, FLORIDA

The research isn't just anecdotal, and it's not just coming from far-away lands. Among the most startling studies on teas was one published by the West's most respected medical authority, the American Medical Association. The study followed more than 40,000 adults for a decade, and at the seven-year follow-up, it found that those who had been drinking five or more cups of tea per day were 26 percent less likely to die of any cause compared with those who averaged less than one cup.

"I WENT FROM A SIZE 20 TO A SIZE 16 IN JUST ONE WEEK, AND I'M ALIVE WITH ENERGY!"

—TRACY DURST, 45, LEWISTOWN, PENNSYLVANIA

Looking for more immediate results? Another study broke participants into two groups, only one of which was put on a green-tea-rich diet. At the end of just 17 days, those who sipped four to five cups of green tea each lost more belly fat than those who did not, according to *The Journal of Nutrition*. And those results last! After 12 weeks, the green tea group had achieved significantly lower body weights and smaller waistlines than those in the control group. Why? Because catechins, the nutrients that give tea its nutritional punch, are so highly effective at boosting metabolism.

"I WASN'T REALLY CONVINCED IT WOULD WORK, BUT I LOST 5 POUNDS IN MY FIRST WEEK!"

—MARGARET MCGRAW, 50, STILLWATER, MINNESOTA

In fact when you begin the 17 D

Japanese researchers found that levels of antioxidants called polymerized polyphenols, found in green tea, inhibit the body's ability to absorb fat by as much as 20 percent. (It's like a get-out-of-jail-free card!) When Taiwanese researchers studied more than 1,100 people over a 10-year period, they determined that those who drank green tea had nearly 20 percent less body fat than those who drank none.

YOU'LL DEACTIVATE THE GENES THAT TRIGGER FAT STORAGE.

Researchers have identified 11 nutrients that turn off fat genes, including those found in fruits, nuts, and eggs. But green tea is unique among foods because it is the best possible source of EGCG, a polyphenol that can deactivate the genetic triggers for diabetes and obesity. Green tea also contains folate, a second critical nutrient that turns off genetic switches for weight gain and insulin resistance.

YOU'LL NEVER FEEL HUNGRY—EVEN AS THE POUNDS MELT AWAY!

EGCG also boosts levels of cholecystokinin, or CCK, a hunger-quelling hormone. In a Swedish study that looked at green tea's effect on hunger, researchers divided up participants into two groups: One group sipped water with their meals, and the other group drank green tea. Not only did tea sippers report less of a desire to eat their favorite foods (even two hours after sipping the brew), they found those foods to be less satisfying.

YOU'LL LOWER YOUR BLOOD PRESSURE.

According to a study in the Archives of Internal Medicine, people who consumed 120 milliliters of tea every day for at least a year had 46 percent lower risk of developing hypertension than those who consumed less.

YOU'LL STRENGTHEN YOUR BONES AND PROTECT YOURSELF FROM INJURY.

Chinese scientists exposed bone cells to catechins and found that the nutrients actually helped the bones grow and slowed the breakdown of bone cells. One of the catechins boosted bone growth by 79 percent. And a 2015 study at Osaka University in Japan found that theaflavin-3 (TF-3), an antioxidant in tea, inhibits the function of an enzyme called DNA methyltransferase, which destroys bone tissue as we age. The study, published in the U.S. journal *Nature Medicine*, found that mice suffering from osteoporosis that were given TF-3 showed recovering levels of bone volume similar to those of healthy mice.

Elma Baron, M.D., the study author.

YOU'LL REDUCE STRESS AND SLEEP BETTER.

You probably already know that chamomile tea can help induce sleep. (There's even a brand called Sleepytime.) But science is showing that teas actually work on a hormonal level to lower our agita and bring peace and slumber. Studies have found that certain teas contain compounds that can actually reduce levels of stress hormones in our bodies, bringing on sleep—and reducing the body's ability to store fat! (In fact, the *17-Day Green Tea Diet* also includes a nightly helping of herbal tea to help reduce your levels of fat-storing stress hormones.)

YOU'LL LOWER YOUR RISK OF CANCER AND OTHER THREATS TO YOUR HEALTH AND HAPPINESS.

A recent study at Penn State found that EGCG triggers a virtuous cycle that kills off cancer cells. "EGCG does something to damage the mitochondria" of cancer cells, says Joshua Lambert, associate professor of food science at Penn State's Center for Plant and Mushroom

INTRODUCTION

Foods for Health. Yet at the same time, it also boosts the protective capabilities of the normal cells surrounding the cancer cells. And a 2015 study from the Institute of Food Research found that the polyphenols in green tea block a "signaling molecule" called VEGF, which in the body can trigger both heart disease and cancer.

So why haven't doctors been touting the benefits of green tea every time you go in for a checkup? Because Western medicine is built around selling you drugs and procedures. If everything from weight gain to diabetes to high blood pressure can be cured with green tea, well, then there's a lot of money to be lost by the hospitals, health clubs, and drug companies.

But there's a lot to be gained by you.

In this book, you'll learn not only about the benefits of green tea but also about how different types of green tea—in particular the powdered variety known as matcha—can improve upon the already proven effects of standard tea, boosting your fat burning and health benefits even more. And you won't ever feel hungry or frustrated. You'll discover the Five Green Superfoods, foods so powerful they will fuel your health, your energy and your weight-loss in the next 17 days and for months to come. In fact, consuming as little as ¼ cup of one of the Green Superfoods daily, in combination with green tea, has been shown to cause dramatic, long-term losses in belly fat in just two weeks. (After 24 weeks, those who ate it experienced a massive 62 percent greater decrease in weight and BMI than standard dieters, according to the journal *Nature*.)

If it all sounds too good to be true, then do yourself this one simple favor: Simply commit to the *17-Day Green Tea Diet* for just a few days. You'll be shocked to see how quickly the needle on the scale starts to move and how loose your pants start to feel. Jeannine Arenas of Miami dropped 9 pounds in just seven days—despite having a thyroid disorder that makes weight loss difficult. Margaret McGraw lost 5 pounds in her first week, while Tracy Durst lost more

THE 17-DAY GREEN TEA DIET

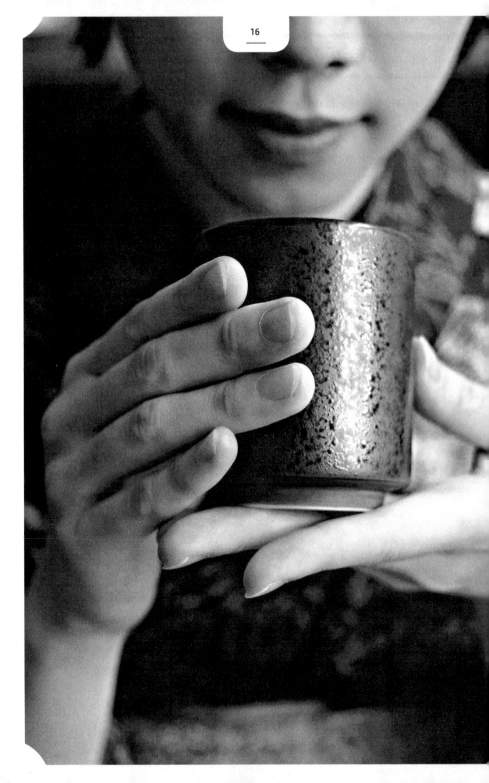

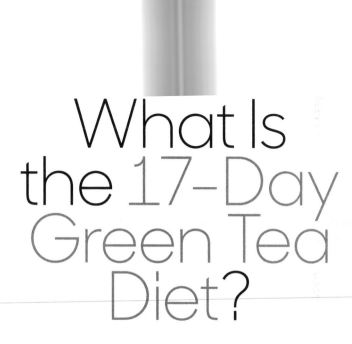

What Is the 17-Day Green Tea Diet?

Discover how four cups of tea plus the Five Green Superfoods can change your life in just 17 days!

WHAT IS THE 17-DAY GREEN TEA DIET?

The *17-Day Green Tea Diet* is unlike any other weight-loss plan you've ever tried. And that's a good thing.

The easiest way to explain this plan might be to tell you what it's not: It's not a low-carb plan that will leave you hungry, grumpy, and standing outside the bakery looking longingly at crave-worthy cakes. It's not a calorie-restriction program that requires you to calculate every bite you take like you're Stephen Hawking looking for a lost planet. And it's not a new gimmick, temporary trend, or questionable concept based on some study of five blind mice in a college laboratory.

In fact, there may be more research proving the effectiveness of green tea than for any other weight-loss plan in human history. And that's in part because certain cultures have been using it for thousands of years to control hunger, improve health, and boost metabolism and performance.

Fortunately, there's never been a better time to immerse yourself in the weight-loss powers of this remarkable drink. A wide variety of green teas are becoming more and more available as Westerners discover their weight-loss powers. In fact, Americans drank 10.7 percent more tea in 2014 than they did in 2012—about 3.6 billion gallons of the stuff, according to the Tea Association of the U.S.A. And the organization predicts that sales will double in just the next five years.

So how can you make this perfectly timed trend work for you?

THE 17-DAY GREEN TEA DIET

son: A study in the International Journal of Molecular Science found that fasting overnight, followed by green tea intake (at least 30 minutes before your first meal of the day), allowed for the best possible absorption of EGCG, the magic nutrient in green tea. Additionally, you'll maximize your EGCG levels by creating a 4½-hour window between lunch and dinner, with a green tea 30 minutes before eating.

There's an added benefit to skipping breakfast: Green tea is proven to increase metabolism, so you'll begin burning body fat early in the morning and keep burning it all day long. To turbocharge that fat melt, you'll start your day with the lightest of workouts, a simple 10-minute walk that will tell your system that it's time to start burning calories. (Although if you want a more rigorous morning workout, you'll find two short but effective plans later in the book.)

You'll also enjoy three delicious meals each day, each with a perfect balance of healthy fats, protein, fiber, and micronutrients: one lunch, one dinner, and a Green Tea Smoothie.

Each meal is based on three or more of the Green Superfoods:

GREEN TEA

Green tea—whether in bags, loose leaf, or powdered like matcha—not only is your go-to drink for melting fat and boosting metabolism but also plays an important role in many of the recipes you'll discover later in this book. And it serves as the foundation of each day's Green Tea Smoothie.

Basing your smoothie on green tea helps ensure that you're always getting a consistent flow of tea-based nutrients, so slimming down becomes automatic. In a study presented at the North American Association of the Study of Obesity, researchers found that regularly drinking smoothies in place of meals increased a person's chances of losing weight and keeping it off longer than a year.

Green Tea Smoothies are designed to be creamy, filling, and packed with protein, fiber, and healthy fats. (You'll read more about those important nutrients below.) And because they're plant-based, these smoothies also help ensure that you're getting a healthy dose of the nutrients most Americans are missing from their diets. Researchers at Baylor College of Medicine found that dieters who drank 8 ounces of plant-based juices a day over a 12-week period lost, on average, 4 pounds more than dieters following the exact same plan but without the drinks. And a Vanderbilt University study found that people who consume three or more servings of fruit- and vegetable-based drinks each week are 76 percent less likely to develop Alzheimer's over a 10-year period than those who don't.

WHAT TO EAT AND DRINK: Four cups of green tea each day, plus one Green Tea Smoothie per day; you'll find recipes in Chapter Eight. Plus, you'll find green tea to be one of the key ingredients in many of the lunch, dinner and snack recipes in that chapter.

... . very few calories. Bright colors signal that the vegetables are rich in polyphenols, micronutrients that help control diet-induced inflammation. And vegetables, especially the leafy kind, have very few calories and a low glycemic load—meaning they load up your body with nutrients without generating a spike in blood sugar.

Research from the University of Otago in New Zealand found that participants felt happier, calmer, and more positive on days when they consumed fruits and vegetables. And further research has identified folate as a critical nutrient for turning off the genes related to insulin resistance and fat storage. A study in the *British Journal of Nutrition* found that those with the highest folate levels lose 8.5 times more weight when dieting. Indeed, some scientists believe that folate level is the primary indicator of a healthy diet; when folate levels drop, levels of obesity, heart disease, stroke, cognitive impairment, Alzheimer's, and depression go up.

WHAT TO EAT: Lettuces and leafy greens like kale, watercress, spinach, and chard; collard greens and beet greens; cabbage, kohlrabi, broccoli, brussels sprouts, and asparagus; and brightly colored vegetables like red peppers, grape tomatoes, carrots, and beets.

GREEN, RED, ORANGE, AND YELLOW FRUITS

To maximize the effectiveness of your green tea, you'll seek out natural sources of vitamin C—and that means plenty of whole, delicious fruit. Studies show that vitamin C may improve EGCG bioavailability by preventing oxidation—a good reason to consider adding a splash of lemon to your tea.

But fruits do more than just improve your EGCG absorption. Green fruits like kiwi get their color from chlorophyll, which helps with the formation of new blood cells and the assimilation of magnesium and calcium; it also helps create a more alkaline body environment. Fruits that come in green and red—apples, grapes, and berries—also have their own particular fat-busting properties. For example, in a recent Texas Women's University study, researchers found that feeding mice three daily servings of berries decreased the formation of fat cells by up to 73 percent. Another study at the University of Michigan found that rats that had berry powder mixed into their meals had less abdominal fat at the end of 90 days than those on a berry-free diet.

Green, red, orange, and yellow fruit can also make you look younger almost overnight: A study in *Evolution and Human Behavior* found that people who ate more of these had a more sun-kissed complexion than those who didn't consume as much, thanks to nutrients called carotenoids. In fact, given the choice between a real suntan and a glow caused by diet, study participants preferred the carotenoid complexion.

Another important nutritional component you'll get from fruit: fiber. A recent study at Wake Forest Baptist Medical Center found that for every 10-gram increase in soluble fiber eaten per day, abdominal fat was reduced by 3.7 percent over five years.

Melons belong on your *17-Day Green Tea Diet* table as well. Research at the University of Kentucky showed that eating watermelon, for

....: If you're selecting which apples to buy, an analysis in the *Journal of Agricultural and Food Chemistry* found that Red Delicious, Northern Spy, Cortland, Ida Red, Golden Delicious, McIntosh, and Macoun were the most nutritious varieties.

GREEN FATS

A green fat is one that comes from green plants like olives and avocados, as well as from trees, in the form of tree nuts and coconut. (Peanuts count, too.) Though it may seem counterintuitive to add fat to a meal if you're trying to lose it, eating a moderate portion of unsaturated fats, like the kind found in olive oil, avocados, and nuts, can ward off the munchies and keep you full by regulating hunger hormones. A study published in *Nutrition Journal* found that participants who ate half a fresh avocado with lunch reported a 40 percent decreased desire to eat for hours afterward.

Changing the kind of fat in your diet will also help you increase your intake of omega-3 fatty acids while reducing omega-6 (found in vegetable oil and fried foods); upping your omega-3-to-6 ratio has been proven to improve metabolic health and reduce inflammation. And according to a study review in the *International Journal of Molecular Science*, omega-3 polyunsaturated fatty acids may enhance not only the bioavailability of EGCG but also its effectiveness.

To improve your fat profile, reduce the amount of fat you take in from grains. So: Say goodbye to vegetable oil (it's not from vegetables!) and to corn, soy, and safflower oils as well. In fact, simply cutting out vegetable oil—which comes primarily from soybeans—can have a massive impact your waistline. A 2015 study at the University of California Riverside found that, in mice at least, a diet high in soybean oil causes more obesity and diabetes than a diet high in sugar. Compared to animals on a coconut-oil diet, the mice that ate sugar gained 9 percent more weight. But the creatures that ate soybean oil gained 25 percent more!

WHAT TO EAT: Avocados and olives; olive oil, canola oil, and gourmet oils like walnut and hazelnut.

GREEN PROTEINS

What, exactly, is a "green protein"? Sounds like something that's been sitting in the back of the fridge for a few months.

By green proteins, we mean one of two things: proteins made from green sources—like nuts and seeds, vegan protein blends, or spirulina—or animals whose diets are primarily green, like grass-fed beef, free-range chicken, or wild fish. Keeping your protein lean and green will also help improve the fat profile of your diet while helping to quell inflammation.

But most important: Eating enough protein is critical to helping EGCG do its job. Studies show that those who have low levels of serum albumin—a type of protein found in the blood—also have lower levels of EGCG. Albumin is essential for moving fluids and nutrients between the bloodstream and the body tissues. Eating enough lean

opposed to one high in carbs, increases satiety by suppressing the hunger-stimulating hormone ghrelin.

The Green Tea Smoothie recipes you'll find in this book are all built around plant-based protein powders—low-sugar, high-fiber alternatives to popular dairy-based supplements. A study by the University of Tampa that compared plant protein with whey found it to be equally as effective at changing body composition and boosting muscle recovery and growth. And in a 2015 study in the *Journal of Diabetes Investigation*, researchers discovered that patients who ingested higher amounts of vegetable protein were far less susceptible to metabolic syndrome (a combination of high cholesterol, high blood sugar, and obesity). A second study in *Nutrition Journal* found that "plant protein intakes may play a role in preventing obesity."

With less sugar and a healthier fat profile, plant-based proteins will also improve your gut health at the same time as they're fueling your muscles. Hemp, rice, and pea proteins are all good options; however, you'll want to ensure you're getting a complete protein with a full amino acid profile, which is why a blend that combines all three is superior.

"Green meats," on the other hand, are fish and animals that eat natural, green foods: wild fish, free-range poultry, and grass-fed beef. Unlike cattle that are fattened up with corn, those raised solely on grass produce meat that is leaner and healthier—and that will help you trim away the pounds. A 3.5-ounce serving of grass-fed beef has only 2.4 grams of fat, compared with 16.3 grams for conventionally raised cattle. Grass-fed beef also has higher levels of healthy omega-3 fatty acids and lower levels of inflammatory omega-6s. (So you're boosting your EGCG levels in two ways!) And it's also higher in both vitamin E and conjugated linoleic acid (CLA), which has been shown to reduce abdominal fat while helping build lean muscle. It's the same with chickens: According to a study in the journal *Poultry Science*, free-range chickens have significantly more omega-3s than grain-fed chickens, less harmful fat, and fewer calories.

And while you might not consider fish as coming from a farm, the fact is that almost all of the salmon, shrimp, and tilapia sold in the U.S. comes from fish farms, where they're fed soy pellets laced with chemicals. That means the heart-healthy benefits of eating fish are actually flopped, and farmed fish aren't at all good for your health. In fact, a study in the *Journal of the American Dietetic Association* warned people who are concerned about heart disease to avoid eating tilapia for just that reason.

Now, given how good protein is for your calorie burn, you may be tempted to grab one of those expensive protein bars instead of sitting down to a decent meal. But the effect isn't the same: Not only are you getting a lot of extra sugar and chemicals, but you're not getting the same fat-fighting effects—studies show that your body burns more calories digesting whole foods than it does digesting processed foods.

WHAT TO EAT: Vegan protein blends (you'll find them in any health-food shop); nuts, seeds, and nut and seed butters; grass-fed beef; free-range pork and poultry; wild-caught fish.

While it's not one of the Five Green Superfoods, make an effort to add some black pepper to your meal whenever it's appropriate. Recent studies have indicated that a compound found in black pepper called piperine may help improve blood levels of EGCG by allowing it to linger in the digestive system longer—meaning that more of it is absorbed by the body.

The 17-Day Green Tea Diet Cheat Sheet

MEALS

Two meals a day: a filling Green Lunch and a delicious Green Dinner. Plus, you'll enjoy a nutrition-packed snack and a dessert-like Green Tea Smoothie.

HOT TEAS

You'll enjoy one nourishing cup of green tea three times a day. By delivering to your body a steady intake of catechins, you'll keep your metabolism revving high, reduce disease-causing inflammation, and actually shrink your fat cells. Plus, you'll enjoy a calming herbal tea before bedtime to reduce stress, improve focus, and ensure better sleep.

TEA SMOOTHIES

Every day, you're going to look forward to enjoying a cool, creamy, and delicious Green Tea Smoothie. These recipes will keep you full while ensuring your body has all the fat-melting nutrients it needs to amp up your weight loss to the max.

MORNING RITUAL

You'll begin every day not with some sort of horrible exercise routine or nose-crinkling potion but with a gentle walk in the sunshine. All

We've included a 10-minute, full-body workout that will add even more speed to your revving metabolism, plus a seven-minute core workout for off days. While exercise isn't a necessary component of this program, the *17-Day Green Tea Diet* sets your body up for maximum fat burn during physical activity—so why not take advantage of it?

RECIPES

Each of the recipes featured in Chapter Eight is based on three or more of the Green Superfoods, so you'll be receiving a constant flow of nutrients that maximize the effectiveness of your EGCG intake.

FOODS TO FOCUS ON

Green tea; green, leafy vegetables; green, red, orange, and yellow fruits; fruit- and nut-based oils; plant-based proteins and grass-fed and free-range meats; black pepper.

FOODS TO AVOID

Sodas, bottled teas, and other drinks containing added sugar; soy and soy-based foods; soy, corn, and "vegetable" oils; conventionally raised meat and dairy; farmed salmon and tilapia.

—
SEVEN WAYS TO MAKE YOUR GREEN TEA WORK HARDER

1
—

KEEP IT DRY AND COOL.

Store tea in a cool, dry place, preferably in a sealed plastic bag to reduce exposure to air, sunlight, and moisture.

2
—

DRINK IT ON AN EMPTY STOMACH.

Green tea that you drink four hours after your last meal, and at least 30 minutes before your next, will be absorbed at the highest possible levels.

3
—

KEEP YOUR PROTEIN LEVELS UP.

Eat lean, green proteins regularly to ensure your blood protein levels facilitate the absorption of EGCG.

...g... ... vitamin C help boost the effectiveness of EGCG.

5

SEEK OUT SEAFOOD.

Omega-3 fatty acids from fish further help enhance the efficacy of EGCG.

6

SPRINKLE ON THE PEPPER.

Black pepper helps slow the elimination of EGCG from your digestive system, leading to higher absorption levels.

7

FILTER YOUR WATER.

Concentrated levels of certain minerals in water can interfere with the absorption of EGCG. If you have hard water, consider using a water filter.

Green Tea: The Next Level

Most of what we think of as green tea comes in tea bags found at the local grocery store. And indeed, store-bought green tea bags are a potent weapon against belly fat. The majority of research cited in this book—and the test-panel results—comes from grocery-store-variety green tea.

But if you're the adventurous type who's interested in taking weight loss to another level, you may want to explore the traditional Japanese green tea known as matcha. Matcha is a powdered green tea that some research indicates may be an even more potent weight-loss weapon. Consider:

- The concentration of EGCG—the superpotent nutrient found in green tea—may be as much as 137 times greater in powdered matcha tea. EGCG can simultaneously boost lipolysis (the breakdown of fat) and block adipogenesis (the formation of new fat cells). One study found that men who drank green tea containing 136 milligrams of EGCG— what you'd find in a single 4-gram serving of matcha—lost twice as much weight than a placebo group and four times as much belly fat over the course of three months.

.... .at-burning benefits of standard green tea are already remarkable, and you'll learn more about them in the coming chapters. But if you want to take your health and weight loss to another level, you'll find directions for making matcha tea in Chapter Four.

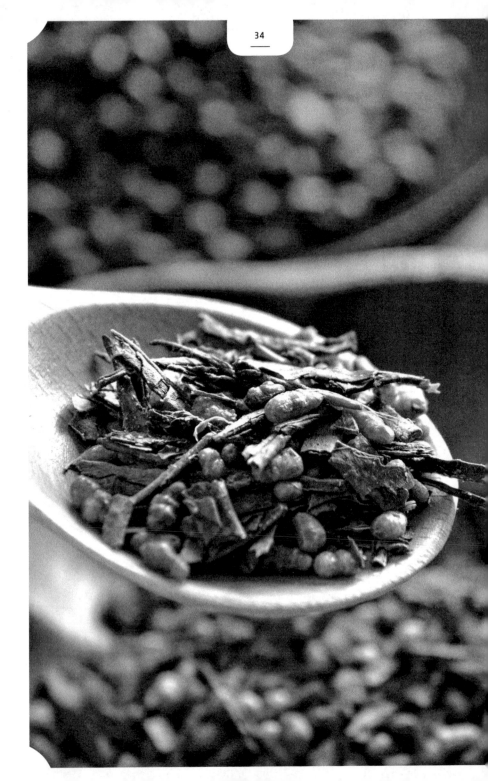

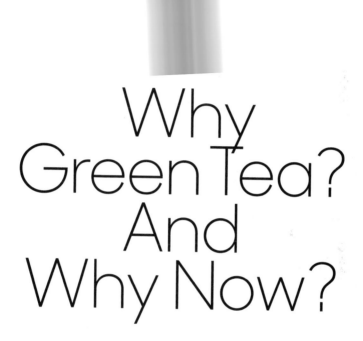

Why Green Tea? And Why Now?

The shocking new science of stripping off the pounds

It seems odd, doesn't it? The airwaves, the Internet, the bookstores—they're all packed with weight-loss plans that promise to strip fat from our bodies and return us to health.

Many involve expensive meal plans or special weight-loss formulas; others require meetings and memberships and confusing point systems; still more are built around challenging workouts and costly gym equipment.

But the humble green tea blows all those programs out of the water, for many reasons.

GREEN TEA DEACTIVATES YOUR FAT-STORAGE GENES.

It's true: Green tea works on your body on a genetic level, turning "off" the genes that are related to fat storage and making weight loss effortless.

If that sounds like science fiction, it's not: It's the new science of nutritional genetics, and it's changing everything we know about weight loss. A 2014 study in the journal *Advanced Nutrition* found that obese and diabetic people have different patterns of gene markers than those who are not obese or diabetic. Essentially, say the researchers, the "on" switches for their fat-storage genes have been tripped. In another review of 46 different studies on the topic of obesity and genetics, researchers writing in the *International Journal of Obesity* in 2014 reported that genetic markers for obesity— evidence that fat genes have been turned on—can be spotted at birth, and those markers can predict whether a newborn will become obese as an adult.

"What you eat, and don't eat, can influence which genes are turned

.... ʋʜaʋ ρɪay a ᴅɪg role in epigenetics, especially folate," say Schalinske.

GREEN TEA BOOSTS YOUR METABOLISM.

Another reason why green tea is the right move, right now, is our further understanding of the importance of increasing one's resting metabolic rate. Basically, years of diet trends—eating nothing but grapefruit or cabbage soup or cottage cheese—have proven only one thing: When you restrict calories, you reset your resting metabolism to "slow." People who lose dramatic amounts of weight by cutting way back on their food intake wind up losing more than fat; they lose muscle as well.

And muscle is a powerful fat burner. In fact, muscle burns energy all day long, just by being there on your body, ready to help with the groceries. It steals energy away from fat cells—specifically belly-fat cells—in order to maintain itself. (Pound for pound, muscle burns three times as many calories as fat does, every single day!)

If you restrict calories in the traditional crash-diet way, your body will react by losing weight, all right. But much of the weight you shed will be muscle. In fact, in a recent study that got a lot of attention, researchers put a group of men on a diet of 360 calories a day and made them exercise for nine hours a day. After four days, the men lost 11 pounds—but the majority of the weight they lost wasn't fat, it was muscle. Green tea, on the other hand, protects your muscles: Brazilian scientists found that participants who consumed three cups of the beverage every day for a week had fewer markers of the cell damage caused by resistance to exercise. That means that green tea can also help you recover faster after an intense workout.

GREEN TEA CAUSES FAT CELLS TO SHRINK.

So how do we inspire our bodies to burn fat, and retain muscle, so that we keep that high-calorie-burning tissue in place even as the flab melts away? That's where green tea comes in. Green tea is the bandit that picks the lock on your fat cells and drains them away, without damaging your muscles. In fact, it seems to make up for even our most unwise dietary choices. In one study, Chinese researchers divided rats into five groups and fed them varying diets over a two-month period. In addition to a control group, there was a group given a high-fat diet with no tea supplementation and three additional groups that were fed a high-fat diet with varying doses of pu-erh tea extract (a fermented type of green tea). The researchers found that the green tea significantly lowered triglyceride concentrations (potentially dangerous fat found in the blood) and belly fat in the high-fat diet groups.

In another study—this one on people—participants who combined a daily habit of four to five cups of green tea each day with a 25-minute workout for 12 weeks lost an average of two more pounds than the non-tea-drinking exercisers. Once again it's the power of the unique catechins found in green tea that can blast adipose tissue by triggering the release of fat from fat cells (particularly in the belly), then speeding up the liver's capacity for turning that fat into energy.

...ney damage. Another study published in the journal *Biological Chemistry* showed that green tea protected the liver from some of the oxidative stress brought on by alcohol. And Purdue University researchers found that drinking tea with dinner may block the absorption of any toxins in your meal—for example, mercury in fish. (In fact, if you're worried about toxins like mercury, then get to know your tuna: Light chunk tuna is lower in mercury content than albacore.) Other low-mercury fish include shrimp, wild salmon, pollack, and catfish. Avoid higher-contaminant fish like Atlantic salmon, swordfish, shark, king mackerel, marlin, and tilefish.

GREEN TEA BOOSTS YOUR IMMUNE SYSTEM.

EGCG has been shown to stop the adenovirus (one of the bugs responsible for colds) from replicating. Start pumping green tea into your system at the first sign of a cold and you should be able to stave off worse symptoms.

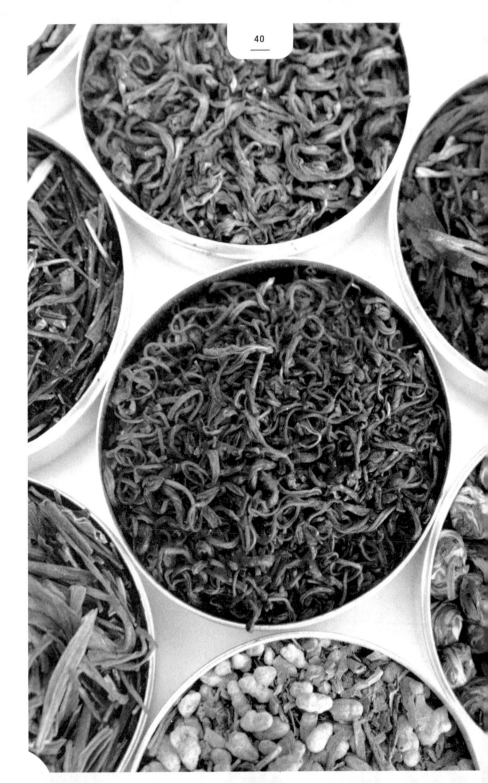

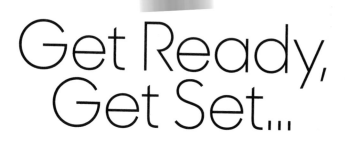

Get Ready, Get Set...

Prepare yourself for rapid weight loss and long-term success

GET READY, GET SET...

If you're like most Americans, when you hear the word tea the first thing that comes to mind is a yellow box from Lipton, or a bottle of Snapple, or a commercial of a guy taking the Nestea plunge. You probably know that green tea is good for you, that a hot tea with honey soothes the throat, and that chai is a flavoring you get at Starbucks.

And that's about it.

But when it comes to our attitude toward tea, we're pretty much alone in the world. From the cold shores of the British Isles to the steamy jungles of Southeast Asia, tea is a critical daily component of many cultures, as ritualized and debated there as craft brews and the NFL draft are here. In many regions, tea leaves are considered as nuanced and diverse as wine grapes. In Japan, an entire formal ceremony is built around the preparation of matcha; in some parts of Great Britain, folks still break at 4 p.m. or so for tea time each day. And like many other cultural rituals, the rituals that formed around tea have a basis in physical and spiritual health. In the coming pages, you'll read more about how to prepare tea and use it as your secret weight-loss weapon.

And the good news is that you don't need to have manservants, a geisha, a special tea hut, or even a pair of white gloves to enjoy the maximum flavor and health benefits of tea. But you should keep a few rules in mind if you want to extract all the weight-loss muscle that tea has to offer.

The full program begins in the next chapter. But first, we want to set you up for maximum success by introducing a simple, effective way to slash unwanted calories from your life and turbocharge your transformation.

You see, part of what makes this plan so effective is that it dramatically slashes the No. 1 source of belly fat in the American diet: liquid calories. We mean the stuff you drink every day: sodas, sweet teas, energy drinks, lattes, juices, and the like.

The averag̲e̲

̲factory. Those three drinks alone give you 920 additional calories—almost half a day's worth!

In fact, liquid calories now make up a whopping 21 percent of our daily calorie intake—more than 400 calories every single day, more than twice as much as we drank 30 years ago. To give you a perspective on those numbers, imagine taking two slices of Pizza Hut Thin 'N Crispy Pepperoni Pizza, tossing them in a blender, and hitting "puree," then drinking the whole thing down. That's 420 calories. Now imagine that the typical American has been doing this every single day for years.

Wow. Disgusting, right?

Yes, but behind those slightly sickening statistics comes some great news. Because if you want to strip away pounds, shrink your belly, and begin to sculpt a leaner, fitter body—while also boosting your health, calming your mind, and fighting back against some of the most significant diseases of our time—just changing what you drink could be all you need.

One study at Johns Hopkins University found that people who cut liquid calories from their diets lose more weight—and keep it off longer—than people who cut food calories. Simply cutting out liquid calories—by switching your usual drink to green tea—could save you nearly 42 pounds this year alone!

So to start tapping into the healing power of the *17-Day Green Tea Diet*, you first have to rid yourself of the liquid toxins your body has been piling up. Here's how to do it:

1 SWEAR OFF SODAS AND BOTTLED TEAS

ANNUAL WEIGHT LOSS: 12 pounds

According to the National Institutes of Health, the third largest source of food calories in the American diet isn't a food at all. It's soda. We get more calories from soda every day than we do from meat, dairy, or anything other than baked goods. How can that be possible? Because of all the sugar. Mountain Dew, for example, not only delivers 52 grams of sugar per 12-ounce can but also gives you a delicious side helping of brominated vegetable oil, a component of rocket fuel. And we don't mean metaphorical rocket fuel—we mean the stuff they actually put in the engines to keep the gears from exploding.

2 DON'T DRINK JUICE DRINKS

ANNUAL WEIGHT LOSS: 19 pounds

If the FDA ever forces drink manufacturers to start properly labeling their products, SunnyD would have to be called ObesiD. (Some versions of the brand have up to 180 calories and 40 grams of sugar per serving.) Most of these "juice" drinks are really just water and high-fructose corn syrup. If you drink just one of these a day, cut it out—you'll lose 19 pounds this year!

..... ⅃ℎe average caloric impact
of the blended drinks was 239 calories. Switch to tea just once a day
and you'd lose 25 pounds this year! (Actually, you may lose more, as
coffee has been linked to belly-fat storage.)

4 USE TEA TO "FLAVOR" YOUR WATER

ANNUAL WEIGHT LOSS: 13½ pounds

In one of the greatest feats of marketing ever, Vitaminwater pro-
duces products that sound a lot like health drinks but are nothing
more than straight-up sugar. Its Power-C Dragonfruit flavored water
has 120 calories and 31 grams of sugar—that's the equivalent of
drinking 13 Jolly Ranchers. You would lose more than a pound a
month just by making this one swap each day.

5 CHOOSE TEA OVER JUICE

ANNUAL WEIGHT LOSS: 14½ pounds

What could be healthier than this: Langers Pomegranate Blueberry
Plus? It's 100 percent juice, says so right on the label. But the "Plus" is
juice concentrate, which is so sweet that Langers packs 30 grams of
sugar in each 8-ounce glass: That's the sugar equivalent of two—
two!—Snicker's Ice Cream Bars.

6 MAKE YOUR OWN ICED TEA

ANNUAL WEIGHT LOSS: 13½ pounds

Once a tea is made and sits on a supermarket shelf for, oh, an entire NFL season, the nutrients have spent enough time exposed to light and air that they begin to break down. Plus, who knows what else has worked its way into that bottle? Snapple's All Natural Green Tea packs 120 calories and 30 grams of sugar, while Ssips Green Tea with Honey & Ginseng is sweetened not so much with honey but with high-fructose corn syrup. In fact, a few years back, the authors of *Eat This, Not That!* commissioned ChromaDex laboratories to analyze 14 different bottled green teas for their levels of disease-fighting catechins. While Honest Tea Honey Green Tea topped the charts with an impressive 215 milligrams of total catechins, some products weren't even in the game. For instance, Republic of Tea Pomegranate Green Tea had only 8 milligrams, and Ito En Teas' Tea Unsweetened Lemongrass Green Tea had just 28 milligrams, despite implying on its label that the product is packed with antioxidants.

Why the discrepancy? The fact is, store-bought bottled teas typically lose 20 percent of EGCG/catechin content during the bottling process, which is why brewing your own is so critical. If you really want bottled tea, then shoot for versions with an acid like lemon juice or citric acid, which helps stabilize EGCG levels. Recent studies show that the more acidic the environment, the more stable the tea's nutrients. But even in a highly acidic drink, more than half of the nutrients are gone within three months.

THE 17-DAY GREEN TEA DIET

Placing SoBe tea in the same book with the
healthy choices in these pages is sort of like posting Charles
Manson's photo among the babysitters at Care.com.
The Pepsi-owned company's flagship line, composed of
11 flavors with names like "Nirvana" and "Cranberry
Grapefruit Elixir," is marketed to give consumers the
impression that it can cleanse the body, mind, and spirit.
Don't be fooled. This bottle of green tea contains
240 calories and 61 grams of sugar—that's the sugar
equivalent of four slices of Sara Lee Cherry Pie.

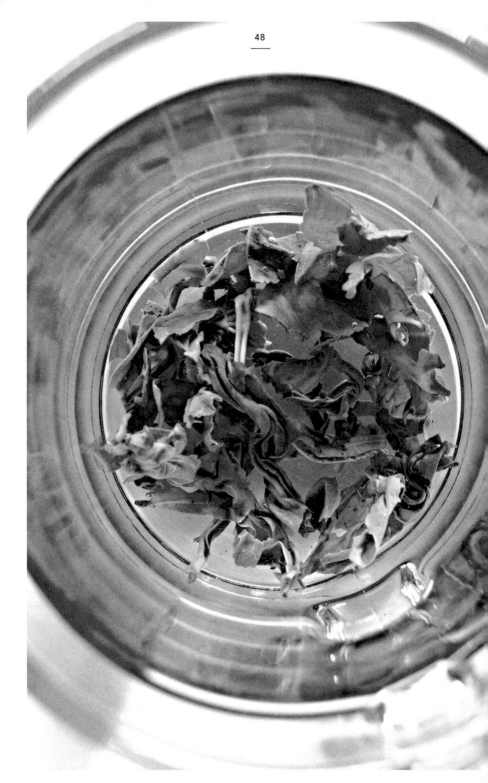

Fat-Blocking Teas

The best teas for shutting down your fat-storage system and telling your fat cells to flake off!

FAT-BLOCKING TEAS

From England to India, Morocco to Japan, tens of millions of people plan their travel and work schedules around tea.

Tea is unique among beverages in that it can be both a private and a social event—a ritual you can enjoy alone before bedtime or with a close girlfriend catching up on the latest gossip. And with the exception of tap water, there's no beverage on earth that's quite as affordable. You don't have to order it from a fancy delivery service, spend oodles of your hard-earned dough on proprietary concoctions, or become a monk who can't join in social events because there's none of your magic elixir on hand. If you have a few dimes and access to hot water, you've got it made. Here's the complete *17-Day Green Tea Diet* program!

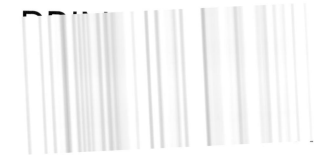

TEAS

You'll enjoy a warm, comforting cup of green tea four times a day, plus a cozy herbal tea of your choice before bedtime. Your first tea of the day will come at least 30 minutes before your first meal to ensure maximum EGCG absorption. You'll also space out lunch, dinner, snacks, and tea consumption in the afternoon to ensure your blood levels of EGCG remain optimized throughout the day.

MEAL PLAN
– all the meals are built around the green superfoods:

GREEN TEA

Many of the recipes in this book incorporate the rich, smoky flavors of green tea. As a cooking broth, an addition to spices and rubs, or a flavoring for desserts, adding green tea into your meals helps to ensure you remain at peak levels of EGCG throughout the day.

GREEN, LEAFY VEGETABLES

On this diet, you'll be focused on getting plenty of folate, the nutrient found primarily in green vegetables and green tea that helps control our body's weight-storage system. In a study of those trying to lose weight, published in the *British Journal of Nutrition*, a 1 nanogram per milliliter increase in serum folate levels increased the chances of weight-loss success by 28 percent.

GREEN, RED, ORANGE, AND YELLOW FRUITS

These fruits tend to be highest in vitamin C, which helps boost the effectiveness of EGCG.

GREEN FATS

A green fat comes from green plants like olives and avocados, as well as from trees, in the form of nuts. Omega-3 fatty acids found in walnuts, chia seeds, flax, and seafood help enhance the efficacy of EGCG.

GREEN PROTEINS

Green proteins are any proteins made from green sources—like vegan proteins or spirulina—or animals whose diets are primarily green, like grass-fed beef, free-range chicken, or wild fish. High-protein foods make EGCG more effective.

GREEN LUNCHES

Consist of a delicious high-protein, high-nutrient, low-calorie meal (under 500 calories) featuring meat, vegetables, whole grains, fruits—all your favorite foods.

GREEN SNACKS

Help bring the benefits of green tea into your day in one more nutritious way. We've identified a variety of snacks that incorporate green tea as part of their makeup or that add powerful nutrients that help make green tea more effective. (How about a Green Tea Panna Cotta?)

> **NOTE:** The average American woman consumes between 1,850 and 2,200 calories every day; the average American man, closer to 2,700. This program brings your daily calorie intake to around 1,300 a day. That calorie deficit alone means the average woman will drop 4 pounds in 10 days just on calories alone—and the average man, about 5. But that's before factoring in the metabolic impact, the debloating power, and the way in which green tea causes fat cells to resist growth. According to the latest research, your results may be as much as 14 pounds in 17 days!

GREEN TEA SMOOTHIES

Every day, you're going to look forward to enjoying a cool, creamy, and delicious Green Tea Smoothie. Just like the smoothies you love from places like Jamba Juice or Smoothie King, these smoothies are a delicious blast of sweet, soothing nutrition. But unlike the ones at those joints, these smoothies will do something very different: They'll strip fat from your body instead of packing it on with obscene sugar counts. Consider this:

At Smoothie King, a 20-ounce Peanut Power Plus Chocolate will cost you 698 calories and 63 grams of sugar. (That's as much sugar as you'll find in 10 chocolate Oreos!) And an Orange Ka-BAM packs 469 calories and 108 grams of sugar. (What you'd get from 43 gummy bears!)

At Jamba Juice, a Strawberry Surf Rider will cost you 450 calories and 98 grams of sugar. (That's 3 full cups of Breyers Vanilla Ice Cream!)

At Starbucks, an Iced White Chocolate Mocha delivers 340 calories and 52 grams of sugar. (That's like having 3½ Snicker's Ice Cream Bars!)

ALCOHOL

No more than one drink every other day, preferably wine. To start with, alcohol is loaded with calories, so cutting down on booze is one of the fastest ways to get rid of empty calories. But alcohol is particularly bad for your weight because it's a toxin. Ingest a beer or a glass of wine and your body mobilizes to burn off the calories in that drink as quickly as possible—ignoring any other calories that might have come along with it. So whether it's wine and cheese or beer and wings, the drink gets metabolized while the body shoves a higher percentage of the accompanying food calories into fat cells.

exercise later in the day. The key is to do a light workout before you eat anything—no latte, no smoothie. The only thing to have beforehand is a cup of green tea, which will help maximize the effects of your workout. Here's why: Once you eat, you give your body a boost of glycogen—the energy that powers your day. So now when you exercise, you need to burn off that glycogen before you start to touch your fat stores. But walk *before* you eat and your burn will come primarily from fat. A study from England's Northumbria University found that people burn up to 20 percent more body fat by exercising in the morning on an empty stomach.

DESSERT

None. By ending your eating by 7 p.m., you'll set yourself up to begin burning fat first thing in the morning. Not just burning calories—burning fat. And your first morning cup—a green tea that jumpstarts your body's internal furnace—will double the effects of your simple fast. Every step you take, every move you make (sorry, Sting), you'll be burning fat.

WORKOUT

Optional. This book concludes with a stunningly effective, metabolism-boosting workout that will rev up the effects of the *17-Day Green Tea Diet* and help you shed belly fat faster than you ever imagined. However, exercise should be considered optional on this program.

The 17-Day Green Tea
Meal Plan

7 am   One to two cups green tea

7:30 am   Morning ritual
(10- to 30-minute walk, preferably outdoors)

10 am   8-ounce Green Tea Smoothie
(at least 30 minutes between last cup and smoothie)

12 pm   Green Superfood Lunch

2 pm   Green Superfood Snack
(if necessary)

3 pm   One cup green tea
(helps control cravings)

6 pm   One cup green tea
(at least four hours between lunch or snack and this cup)

6:30 pm   Green Superfood Dinner
(at least 30 minutes between last cup and dinner)

9 pm   One cup herbal tea
(kava kava, ashwagandha, passionflower, hops, rooibos,
lemon balm, valerian, chamomile with lavender)

... also isn't a good cup of tea, at least according to aficionados and health experts. By tweaking your tea ever so slightly, you can ensure you're getting maximum flavor and maximum health benefits. Here's how:

CONSIDER INVESTING IN LOOSE TEA LEAVES. While tea bags are the cheapest, fastest, and most convenient ways to get your tea fix, a report by ConsumerLab.com, an independent site that tests health products, found that green tea brewed from loose tea leaves yielded the highest levels of EGCG. The report compared a single teaspoonful of Teavana's Gyokuro green tea with single bags of green tea sold by Lipton and Bigelow. Researchers found that the loose green tea yielded about 250 milligrams of catechins, while the tea bags yielded slightly less. But loose tea is more expensive: The report calculated that to obtain 200 milligrams of EGCG you'd spend between 27 and 60 cents using tea bags versus $2.18 using loose tea leaves. In addition, folic acid, a B vitamin found in green tea that also helps the body resist weight gain and diabetes, is found in high quantities in both loose and bagged teas. But a study in the *Journal of the American Dietetic Association* found that tea bags themselves can inhibit the transfer of folic acid.

GET YOUR MATCHA ON. Matcha is a form of green tea that

→ uses the entire leaf in powdered form, rather than flakes of leaves. Matcha is a ceremonial tea that is gaining in popularity and becoming more widely available. Because the powdered tea dissolves directly into the water (and you can brew it hot or cold), some believe that a greater percentage of the nutrients in matcha become available to your body than with standard green teas. Some studies have shown the concentration of EGCG in matcha to be 137 times greater than the amount you'll find in most store-bought green tea. EGCG is a dieter's best friend; studies have shown the compound can simultaneously boost lipolysis (the breakdown of fat) and block adipogenesis (the formation of fat cells), particularly in the belly. One study found that men who drank green tea containing 136 milligrams of EGCG—what you'll find in a single 4-gram serving of matcha—lost twice as much weight than a placebo group and four times as much visceral (belly) fat over the course of three months. Be aware that there are different grades of matcha; while China is now producing this product to varying degrees of success, the best matcha comes from Japan and will be a bright green. Knockoffs may be brownish and bitter. (See "The Matcha Tea Ritual" for traditional brewing instructions.)

TRY GOING PU-ERH. Pu-erh is a type of green tea that's fermented and comes in little green balls that look a bit more like contraband you'd buy at a Phish show than like typical tea. Animal studies have shown that pu-erh decreases fat storage and helps regulate blood sugar levels. Among humans, it's been shown to have anti-cancer properties. And in China, pu-erh is considered a traditional hangover remedy.

HIT THE RIGHT TEMPERATURE. When the teakettle blows, take the water off the heat and let it rest for about 30 seconds, says

...ﬧﬧ ﬩ﬧ ﬧﬧ green tea) before you add it to your tea leaves. If using more potent pu-erh tea, you can use water that's boiling hot.

KNOW YOUR BREW TIMES. A study in the *Journal of Agricultural Food Chemistry* looked at six popular brands of tea and demonstrated that with each type of tea, there is a careful balance between getting the maximum level of nutrients and turning the tea bitter. "The difference between a really good cup and not is to remember to take the leaves out," says Smith. "If you leave them in too long, the cup becomes too strong." Green teas need two to three minutes of steeping time—less than black and mate teas (three to five minutes) or white teas (up to five minutes).

USE A LITTLE LEMON TO MAXIMIZE YOUR BENEFITS. When you sip tea, a significant percentage of the polyphenol antioxidants break down before they reach your bloodstream. But researchers at Purdue University discovered that adding lemon juice to the equation helped preserve the polyphenols.

DITCH THE DAIRY. A study in the *European Heart Journal* found that while tea can improve blood flow and blood-vessel dilation (and thereby lower your blood pressure), adding milk to the tea counteracts these effects.

The Matcha Tea Ritual

Matcha tea has been used in Japanese tea ceremonies since A.D. 1191. Now it's being incorporated into everything from lattes to chocolate to milk shakes.

You can mix this superfood up using just a teacup and a spoon, but it tends to get clumpy and hard to drink. If you want to try making it the traditional way—and unleash a potent brew that's more than 100 times as powerful as standard green tea—here's how:

→ Whisk it up. You don't steep this tea—it's gyokuro green tea that's been ground into a fine powder and whisked with hot water to create a full-bodied, verdant elixir. To make it in the traditional manner, you will need a handmade bamboo whisk (called a chasen), a tea bowl (matcha chawan), a measuring ladle (chashaku), a tea strainer, a teacup, and your matcha powder.

→ To brew a cup, scoop 1½ teaspoons matcha powder into your strainer. Next, sift your matcha powder into your tea bowl, swirling the powder around the strainer with your ladle. This will ensure there are no clumps so your tea will be smooth.

→ Pour boiling water (about 2 ounces) into a teacup, then let it sit until it cools down to about 180 to 190 degrees (about a minute). Carefully pour the hot water into the bowl with the matcha powder.

→ Using your chasen, whisk to combine your tea. Relax your wrist, then whisk in a gentle circular motion for thin, smooth tea or in a brisk M- or W-shaped motion for foamy tea. (Fun fact: Smooth and foamy tea both have slightly different scents and flavors.) Whisk for about 10 to 15 seconds, or until the tea is bright green, then carefully pour your matcha into a teacup. Make sure to drink it right after you've prepared it—the powder will settle at the bottom after a while.

HERBAL STRESS RELIEF

What if we told you that the biggest contributor to your weight gain wasn't sugary drinks, or too much couch time, or the 1,800-calorie Bloomin' Onion you ate the last time you visited Outback? What if the real culprit was something more sneaky and insidious, something you couldn't see, couldn't taste, and couldn't get out of your life? We're talking about stress.

Stress causes fat gain in several different ways:

The stress-nosh effect. You're anxious/bored/worried/ tired, and you need something to occupy your hands/your mouth/the empty feeling in your gut, so you automatically reach for a cookie/ brownie/slice of cake/entire bag of Doritos. Stress drives us to distraction, and distracted eating is eating that adds a lot more calories but few, if any, quality nutrients or feelings of satisfaction.

The fat-storage effect. When you're under stress, the hormone cortisol gathers up all the extra lipids in your bloodstream and stores them right in your belly. Then it sends out a signal: "Hey, need more lipids here. Go eat something." More stress leads to more belly fat, even if actual calories consumed remain the same.

The sleeplessness effect. Sitting up all night long because you can't stop thinking about your credit report, your kids'

loss by cleansing your body of stress and preparing for a night of refreshing, blissful sleep. The following teas can help soothe the soul, bring calm and focus to your world, and improve the quality of your sleep, even on evenings when the gap between income in and payments out is looking precariously narrow.

THE SLEEP ENHANCER
VALERIAN TEA

DRINK THIS: Yogi Tea Herbal Tea Supplement, Bedtime

BECAUSE IT: Brings on deeper sleep

Valerian is an herb that's long been valued as a mild sedative, and now research is showing what tea enthusiasts have known for centuries. In a study of women, researchers gave half the test subjects a valerian extract and half a placebo. Thirty percent of those who received valerian reported an improvement in the quality of their sleep, versus just 4 percent of the control group. In a study published in the *European Journal of Medical Research*, investigators gave 202 insomniacs valerian or a Valium-like tranquilizer. After six weeks, both treatments were equally effective. And in other studies, valerian root has been shown to increase the effectiveness of sleeping pills. While researchers have yet to identify the exact active ingredient, they suspect that receptors in the brain may be stimulated to hit "sleep mode" when coming in contact with valerian.

THE BLUES BUSTER
CHAMOMILE & LAVENDER TEA

DRINK THIS: Traditional Medicinals Organic Chamomile with Lavender

BECAUSE IT: Reduces fatigue and depression

Here's the funny thing about chamomile: While it's the most popular tea for bedtime, there's actually no evidence that it improves the length or quality of sleep. But there's a lot of evidence that it does something even more mysterious: It reduces the stress that comes with insomnia. One German study found that chamomile tea significantly improved the physical symptoms related to a lack of sleep and even helped reduce levels of depression in the chronically sleep-deprived. Another study found that it improved daytime wakefulness in people who suffered from a lack of sleep. To maximize its effects, look for a chamomile/lavender blend. In a study of postpartum women, those who drank lavender tea for two weeks showed improvement in postpartum depression and reduced fatigue. They also reported being able to better bond with their infants.

THE INSOMNIA SLAYER
LEMON BALM

DRINK THIS: Traditional Medicinals Organic Lemon Balm

BECAUSE IT: Reduces sleep disorders

A European study found that lemon balm serves as a natural sedative, and researchers reported that they observed reduced levels of sleep disorders among subjects using lemon balm versus those who were given a placebo.

...activity is due primarily to the bitter resins in the leaves. Hops increase the activity of the neurotransmitter gamma-aminobutyric acid, or GABA, which soothes the central nervous system. Spanish researchers reported in a 2012 journal that the sedative activity of hops aids nocturnal sleep.

THE STRESS-HORMONE SQUASHER
ROOIBOS

DRINK THIS: Celestial Seasonings, Teavana
BECAUSE IT: Reduces cortisol levels

What makes rooibos tea particularly good for soothing your mind is the unique flavonoid called aspalathin. Research shows this compound can reduce stress hormones that trigger hunger and fat storage and are linked to hypertension, metabolic syndrome, cardiovascular disease, insulin resistance, and type-2 diabetes.

THE ANXIETY STOPPER
PASSIONFLOWER

DRINK THIS: Yogi Tea Herbal Tea Supplement, Bedtime
BECAUSE IT: Induces sleepiness and aids anxiety

Passionflower has the flavone chrysin, which has wonderful antianxiety benefits and, in part, can work similarly to the pharmaceutical Xanax (alprazolam). A mild sedative, this particular species of passionflower provides a vegetal-tasting tea that calms nervousness and anxiety and helps you get to sleep at night. It is generally considered safe to use but should be avoided by pregnant women.

THE PERSPECTIVE CHANGER
ASHWAGANDHA

DRINK THIS: Yogi Tea Herbal Tea, Sweet Tangerine Positive Energy

BECAUSE IT: Gives you a better outlook on life

A study in the *Indian Journal of Psychological Medicine* found that "ashwagandha root extract safely and effectively improves an individual's resistance toward stress and thereby improves self-assessed quality of life." In another study, serum cortisol levels in a group of ashwagandha drinkers were substantially reduced versus a placebo group. The plant is used in traditional ayurvedic medicine to treat nervous exhaustion, insomnia, and loss of memory.

THE MIND QUIETER
KAVA KAVA

DRINK THIS: Yogi Tea Herbal Tea, Kava Stress Relief

BECAUSE IT: Quells worrying thoughts

It's one thing to simply sedate. But unlike other teas studied, kava kava actually reduces anxiety levels by helping you get a healthier perspective on life. In one study, 120 milligrams of kava kava were administered daily over six weeks to patients who had stress-induced insomnia. The results suggested a statistically significant improve-

THE 17-DAY GREEN TEA DIET

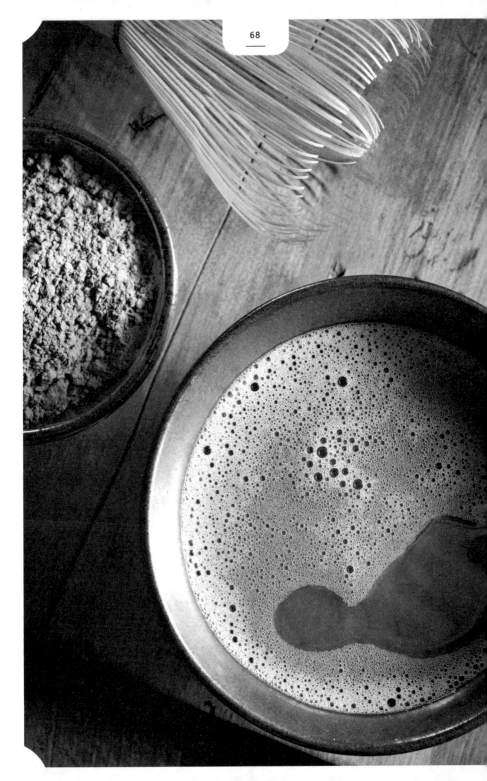

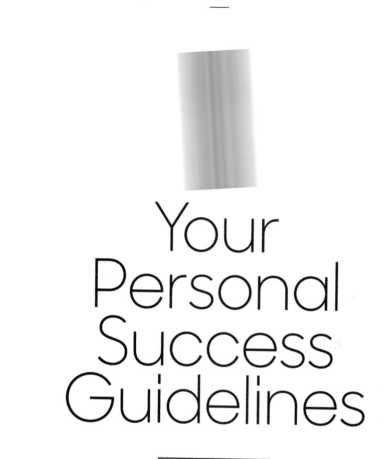

Your Personal Success Guidelines

A mental and emotional preparedness guide for maximum weight-loss success

YOUR PERSONAL SUCCESS GUIDELINES

There's no easier job in the world than selling the promise of a flat belly.

It's like opening a lemonade stand in the Sahara or marketing vanity mirrors to the Kardashians. Lose weight, look great, and have a lean, ripped stomach? Yeah, we'll take that. Who wouldn't?

But if getting rid of body fat is something we all want, why do so few of us take the steps we need to get there? Why do so many of us start on diet or exercise programs, make a little bit of progress, and then fall off? Why does the average weight-loss resolution evaporate after less than three months? And why does even a modest 17-day plan sometimes seem daunting?

Because when it comes to losing weight, vanity is what drives most of us to act. Vanity will get us jump-started every time. But vanity is a terrible long-term motivator. In a study published in 2011 in the *American Journal of Preventive Medicine*, 203 women were enrolled in a six-month weight-loss program at a university weight-loss center. They were divided into three groups. Researchers motivated one group by emphasizing how important weight loss would be to their health. Another, they gave a balanced emphasis of both health and appearance. And the third group, they just focused on how great they were going to look in a bikini at the end of the trial. Guess who lost the most weight?

The bikini group!

While researchers didn't speculate on why the subjects thought jiggling in the wrong places was a worse fate than, say, keeling over clutching their chests, they did conclude that if you want to motivate people to lose weight, then you have to emphasize the vanity aspect.

So vanity is a great way to start: If you found out that you were going to appear on national television in a swimsuit, and you had four weeks to get ready for it, believe us, you'd be pretty motivated to start eating differently—and to stick to it. Nothing is more terrifying

...go, and that cozy couch are right here, right now.

Vanity and fear are two very similar, deeply intertwined emotions. You see a rhino charging straight at you, and fear hits you right in the gut. You want to get out of there—fast. You go to a pool party and feel uncomfortable with how your body looks, and it's a very similar feeling. It hits you right in the gut, and you just want to get out of there—fast.

So the *17-Day Green Tea Diet* is designed to strip away body fat fast—to replace flabby flesh with a lean, toned, sexy physique that will make your partner swoon, fill your friends with envy, and draw the paparazzi to your Jacuzzi. When you walk in the room, heads will swivel, jaws will drop, and plants will turn their leaves to soak up your radiance.

But...

The *17-Day Green Tea Diet* can do more than just whittle your waist. It can change your entire life. See, the reason why most diet and exercise programs fail is the same reason why fleeing a charging rhino won't turn you into a marathon runner. Like fear, vanity can also make us act in fast, decisive, sometimes panicked and irrational ways. But once the initial adrenalin rush is past, we tend to slide back into our old habits.

And that's exactly the trap this program is designed to help you avoid. Losing weight and getting fit are just the tip of the iceberg; the *17-Day Green Tea Diet* will pay off for you in so many ways beyond just how you're going to look. As you begin to see the weight fall away, it's time to think seriously about all the other great benefits you'll gain if you stick with this program. For example:

GREEN TEA WILL MAKE YOU SMARTER!

For years, scientists have understood that midlife obesity is a risk factor for dementia later in life. Just as belly fat helps cause the formation of plaque in your coronary arteries, so, too, does it clog up the arteries feeding the brain—a contributing factor in the development of Alzheimer's. According to researchers at Rush University Medical Center, the protein responsible for metabolizing fat in the liver is the same protein found in the hippocampus, the part of the brain that controls memory and learning. (And that's why EGCG is so critical for all-around health; by helping heal and protect the liver from fat, it also helps protect your brain power.) People with higher levels of abdominal fat actually have depleted levels of this fat-metabolizing protein, making them 3.6 times more likely to suffer from memory loss and dementia later in life.

But a few years ago, scientists discovered something even more ominous. They performed CT scans on a number of healthy middle-aged men and women to measure their visceral fat. What they learned was that the more visceral fat people had, the less brain mass they had.

..., over-the-counter and prescription medicines, and the like) than healthy-weight women. In fact, by one estimate, obesity-related health care will cost Americans $190 billion this year alone.

But the real cost of being overweight doesn't come in the form of prescription pills and diet products. It's not the money we spend; it's the money we don't make. In a study published in the *International Journal of Obesity*, researchers gave participants a series of résumés with small photos of the applicants attached. What they learned was that starting salary, leadership potential, and hiring decisions were impacted negatively when the photo showed a person who was over-weight—most severely in the case of obese women. One study by researchers at the University of Florida found that the thinnest women make a whopping $22,283 more than their overweight peers. For American women, gaining 25 pounds results in an average salary loss of $15,572. Think of it this way: An overweight woman who works for 25 years will wind up with $389,300 less than a thinner one. Add in 25 years of paying that extra eight grand in health care costs, and the total swing between slender and stocky amounts to $598,425. Think dropping 25 pounds might be worth a cool 600 G's?

GREEN TEA WILL IMPROVE YOUR LOVE LIFE!

In studies, women with excess abdominal fat have been shown to have elevated secretions of cortisol, a stress hormone, and an increased sensitivity to stress hormones in the hypothalamus, pituitary, and adrenal glands. Cortisol makes us gain belly fat, so more belly fat equals more cortisol, which equals more belly fat—a nasty cycle. But worse, women who show an increase in cortisol in response to sexual stimuli have lower levels of functioning in certain areas of their sex lives compared with women who show a decrease in cortisol. Good sex comes from less stress. Abdominal fat causes more stress, which causes bad sex.

17-Day Green Tea Diet, are near miracle drugs when it comes to managing your mood. Low levels of folate have been linked to depression, low energy levels, and even memory loss, and studies show that adding folate-rich foods like green tea reduces fatigue, improves energy levels, and helps battle depression. And in a review of studies published in the *American Journal of Psychiatry,* researchers found that deficits in omega-3 fatty acids are a contributing factor in mood disorders; in fact, they speculate that omega-3s may be the common link between heart disease and depression, which tend to run hand-in-hand. And new research published in the British journal *Age and Ageing* indicates that losing belly fat may be the most significant thing you can do to improve your life as you get older. In a study, researchers surveyed nearly 600 men between the ages of 60 and 74, asking them about a wide range of issues, from their physical health to their social lives to their mental and emotional well-being. What they discovered was that the greatest single factor impacting quality of life was belly fat—the more belly fat these men had, the more likely they were to report unhappiness with their lives.

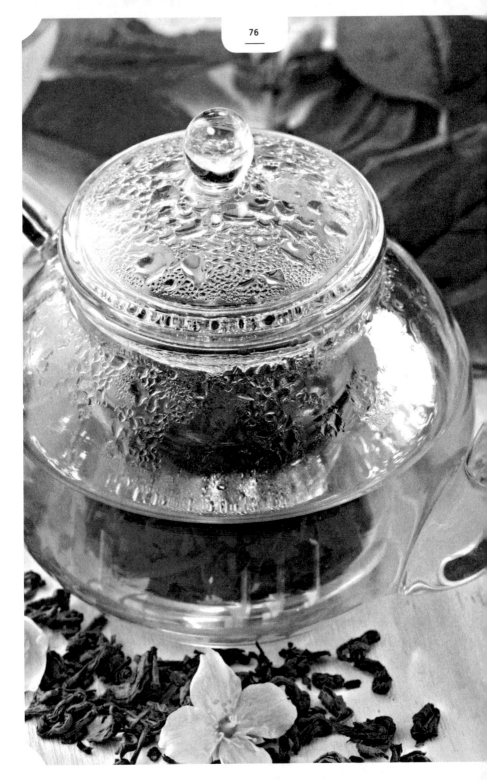

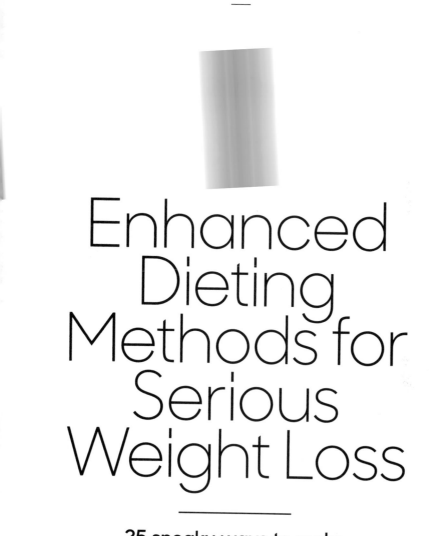

Enhanced Dieting Methods for Serious Weight Loss

25 sneaky ways to make the 17-Day Green Tea Diet **even more effective**

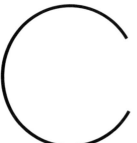ontinue to eat whatever you want, but add green tea to your day, and you will lose weight.

Swap out one of your meals for a Green Tea Smoothie, add green tea to your day, and eat whatever else you want, and you will lose more weight.

Follow the *17-Day Green Tea Diet* protocol and our recipes, and you will lose even more.

And add the *17-Day Green Tea Diet* Workout on top of it all, and your body will react in ways you never thought possible, sculpting itself into a solid tower of lean, healthy, sexy strength.

Such is the power of green tea to boost metabolism, block fat-cell formation, force lipids out of the body, and reduce inflammation that weight loss will become almost automatic, just by adding this miracle drink to your daily food intake. The closer you adhere to the principles of the *17-Day Green Tea Diet*, the more rapid and dramatic your weight loss will become.

But there are tricks to turning the dial up just a tiny bit more. In this chapter, we take a look at some of the tweaks that fitness and nutrition experts use when they want to bring their physiques to the absolute peak of leanness.

DIET ENHANCER 1
DITCH THE GUM

Chewing gum—especially the sugarless kind—may seem like a harmless habit, but one too many sticks can give a whole new meaning to the phrase "bubble butt." Sugarless gums typically contain sorbitol, a sugar alcohol known for causing bloating and other gastrointestinal distress. Sugar alcohols take a relatively long time to digest, and whatever's undigested sits in your small intestine, where it acts as a hothouse for the fermentation of bacteria, causing bloating and flatulence.

̶E̶A̶T̶ ̶P̶O̶P̶C̶O̶R̶N̶
−LEFT-HANDED

We're not suggesting a movie theater binge, but without the butter and excess salt, popcorn can be an apple-shaped snacker's best friend. At only 30 calories, a cup of popped kernels provides more than 9 grams of whole grains—a dietary staple of people with the littlest middles. A Tufts University study found that participants who ate three or more servings of whole grains (oats, quinoa, brown rice) had 10 percent less belly fat than people who ate the same amount of calories from refined carbs (white stuff: bread, rice, pasta). And to keep calories down while you're snacking, consider eating with your non-dominant hand. In a study in the journal *Personality and Social Psychology Bulletin*, moviegoers ate less of a snack when they were prompted to eat only with their non-dominant hands.

DIET ENHANCER 3
USE SMALLER BOWLS

Grabbing handfuls from the bag is never a good idea, but munching from a punch bowl won't do much for weight loss, either. Research in The *FASEB Journal* suggests that overeating may be associated with the size of our serveware. Participants who were given larger bowls served and ate 16 percent more than those given smaller bowls. Not only that, the big-bowlers underestimated just how much they were eating by 7 percent!

DIET ENHANCER 4
IGNORE THE (FRONT) LABEL

Just because something is marketed as "low fat" doesn't mean it's good for you—or you should eat more of it. A Cornell University study in the *Journal of Marketing Research* suggests that people will eat more of a snack that's marketed as "low fat." Participants in the study ate a whopping 28 percent more of a snack (M&Ms!) labeled "low fat" than when they didn't have the label.

DIET ENHANCER 5
COLOR-CODE YOUR SNACKS

A recent study suggests that you can avoid a mindless binge by adding visual traffic lights to your snack. Researchers at the University of Pennsylvania and Cornell University gave one set of students bowls of uniform yellow chips, while another group had their regular snacks layered with differently colored chips. Students who had their snacks segmented ate 50 percent less than those with uniform bowls.

DIET ENHANCER 6
MAKE CINNAMON YOUR NEW FRIEND

Adding a heaping teaspoon of cinnamon to a starchy meal—like sweet potatoes—may help stabilize blood sugar and ward off insulin spikes that can lead to hunger, cravings, and weight gain, according to a series of studies printed in *The American Journal of Clinical Nutrition*.

...buying a brand with the thickening agent carrageenan. Derived from seaweed, carrageenan has been linked to ulcers, inflammation, and other gastrointestinal problems.

DIET ENHANCER 8
INDULGE IN DARK CHOCOLATE

It's every chocoholic's dream: Research now shows that eating moderate amounts of dark chocolate can reduce overall body fat and shrink the waist. A study among women with normal weight obesity who ate a Mediterranean diet that included two servings of dark chocolate each day showed a significant reduction in waist size than when on a cocoa-free meal plan. Researchers say it has to do with the flavonoids, heart-healthy compounds in chocolate that have important antioxidant and anti-inflammatory properties. Just be sure you're reaching for a bar with at least 70 percent cacao, and stay away from the "alkalized" stuff, which has a significantly reduced flavonoid content.

DIET ENHANCER 9
TRY BREAKFAST FOR A SNACK

A quick snack that will fill you up when the weather turns nippy: a bowl of instant oatmeal. Oats are rich in beta-glucan, a form of soluble fiber that acts like your body's LDL bouncer, grabbing bad cholesterol trying to sneak into your system and kicking it to the curb. In a study published in *The American Journal of Clinical Nutrition*, men who ate oat cereal over the course of 12 weeks had lower concentrations of LDL cholesterol than those who were given wheat cereal. Another study printed in the journal *Nutrition* found that the cholesterol-stabilizing power of oatmeal doubled when it was combined with vitamin C—the result of organic compounds called phenols. Top your oats with fresh berries or a small freshly squeezed glass of citrus, and you've got yourself a powerful antidote to elevated cholesterol levels.

DIET ENHANCER 10
DON'T TAKE VITAMINS

Increased levels of B vitamins have long been associated with a higher prevalence of obesity and diabetes. Researchers believe that fortified infant formula at a young age may trigger the fat genes to switch on. If you're more comfortable taking a daily multivitamin, it's probably fine, but megadosing may do more harm than good. Look to get your B vitamins, especially folate, from the Green Superfoods.

. .. containers and also in
the thin plastic linings of food cans. Research has indicated that it may have an epigenetic effect on humans. BPA leaks into foods that are acidic or fatty, like tomatoes, tuna, and baby formula. BPA is used by most manufacturers, but Eden Organic and Trader Joe's both sell BPA-free canned goods.

DIET ENHANCER 12
CUT DOWN ON ANTIBIOTICS

Our gut bacteria play a big role in keeping our fat genes in check by chomping on fiber and creating short-chain fatty acids (SCFAs) such as butyrate, which help tame our genetic propensity for weight gain and diabetes. When we take antibiotics for every sniffle that comes along, we create disorder in our gut bacteria and undermine their ability to create the SCFAs that keep our fat genes in check.

DIET ENHANCER 13
DON'T FEAR THE STARCH

Say the word *starch* to most diet gurus and their heads will start to spin. But "resistant starch" has become one of the big buzz terms in nutrition right now, for good reason. Resistant starch has great metabolism-boosting properties—in fact, it hits both ends of the metabolism spectrum, slowing down your digestive process (thereby

METHODS FOR SERIOUS WEIGHT LOSS

controlling blood sugar), while also forcing your body to burn more calories during the digestion process. But resistant starch has another awesome belly-flattening property: It feeds your gut's "good" bacteria. According to a 2015 study in the *Journal of Functional Foods*, when you eat resistant starch, your gut biome gets stronger—healthy bacteria literally get a workout digesting the healthy starch, becoming more dominant and leading to a healthier gut. Beans, sweet potatoes, bananas, and whole grains like oats and quinoa are among the best sources.

DIET ENHANCER 14
UNFRIEND FACEBOOK

Use of social networks and high Internet use exacerbate feelings of loneliness, and loneliness is the ultimate fat feeling. A new study in the journal *Hormones and Behavior* found that those who feel lonely experience greater circulating levels of the appetite-stimulating hormone ghrelin after they eat, causing them to feel hungrier sooner. Over time, folks who are perennially lonely simply take in more calories than those with stronger social-support networks.

DIET ENHANCER 15
VOLUNTEER

"Because I'm bored" is one of the top reasons people give when they're asked about their emotions before they eat. When you're bored you actually lose your ability to make smart food choices; you become an "emotional eater," according to a new study in the *Journal of Health Psychology*. Boredom stems from feeling dissatisfied, restless, and unchallenged, according to a study in *Frontiers in Psychology*. The best way to beat boredom is to find something to do that is purposeful ...

... only one who gets jet lag when you travel: It turns out our gut microbes have a circadian rhythm, too. A recent study in the journal *Cell* found that our gut microbes are just as affected by changes to our circadian clock as we are. When we shift our sleep/wake cycles our gut flora changes, and beneficial bacteria are replaced by the growth of bacteria that have been linked to obesity and metabolic disease.

DIET ENHANCER 17
REHYDRATE REGULARLY!

In one University of Utah study, diet participants who were instructed to drink two cups of water before each meal lost 30 percent more weight than their thirsty peers. And you can magnify the slimming effects of H2O by adding ice. German researchers found that six cups of cold water a day could prompt a metabolic boost that incinerates 50 daily calories. That's enough to shed 5 pounds a year!

DIET ENHANCER 18
KEEP REGULAR SLEEP HOURS

A recent study found subpar sleep could undermine your weight-loss efforts by as much as 55 percent. The problem: your hormones. Inadequate or broken sleep can throw hunger-regulating hormones out of balance. Ghrelin, the "I'm hungry" hormone, shoots up; leptin, the "I'm full" hormone, decreases. If you have trouble sleeping through the night, stop drinking caffeine after midday, limit your alcohol consumption (which ruins sleep quality), and create a pre-bed ritual to get your body and mind ready for sleep (that doesn't include backlit devices like your TV or tablet). In a recent study, researchers analyzed more than 500 participants' weekday sleep diaries and found that losing a mere 30 minutes of shut-eye increased their risk of obesity by 17 percent.

DIET ENHANCER 19
FLOSS

If your gums bleed when you brush or floss, you could have gingivitis or periodontitis, an inflammation of the gums or around the teeth. And that inflammation isn't just localized within your mouth. Bad bacteria can gain a foothold throughout your digestive system—a condition known as "leaky gut." When your body is chronically inflamed, your internal hormonal communication system can get thrown out of whack, leading to imbalances in your metabolism. Chronic inflammation has been linked to weight gain, insulin resistance, diabetes, and obesity.

DIET ENHANCER 20
GREEN UP YOUR BATHROOM

Most soaps, lotions, and deodorants contain phthalates, listed in the ingredients as "fragrance." These industrial chemicals are also used to make plastics like polyvinyl chloride (PVC) more flexible. They're found in air fresheners, vinyl shower curtains, vinyl flooring, wall coverings, detergents, nail polish, hair spray, shampoo, and other

DIET ENHANCER 21

DROP BY CHIPOTLE

But make sure what you're ordering is rich in beans. Beans are high in the chemical butyrate, which encourages the body to burn fat as fuel. According to a study at the Wake Forest Baptist Medical Center, beans are rich in soluble fiber and can lessen the accumulation of body fat: For each 10 grams of soluble fiber that study subjects added to their diets, they lost 3.7 percent of belly fat in a year!

DIET ENHANCER 22

MAKE QUINOA YOUR GO-TO GRAIN

According to a study published in the journal *Food Chemistry*, quinoa has the highest level of betaine, a chemical that revs your metabolism and actually shuts down the genes that encourage belly fat to hang around. If you find yourself needing some variety, don't turn back to brown rice—look to quinoa's good-carb cousins such as bulgur and barley.

DIET ENHANCER 23
TURN UP THE AC

And make more brown fat! A recent study published in the journal *Diabetes* found that exposure to cold temperatures at night can actually stimulate the growth of calorie-burning brown fat (a good-for-you type of body fat). Researchers from the National Institute of Diabetes and Digestive and Kidney Diseases had participants spend a few weeks sleeping in bedrooms with varying temperatures: a neutral 75 degrees, a cool 66 degrees, and a balmy 81 degrees. After four weeks of sleeping at 66 degrees, the subjects had almost doubled their volumes of brown fat. (And yes, that means they lost belly fat.)

DIET ENHANCER 24
GET ON A ROLL

Foam rolling is one of the best ways to keep your muscles loose and your body mobile. It not only stretches areas that are hard to hit otherwise (like long tendons) but also provides a "dynamic" stretch, meaning one in which you're moving. A recent study found that high-intensity dynamic stretching improves strength and flexibility. Slow, relaxed stretching, not so much.

...gut health (and a shrinking belly), you want to eat prebiotic foods—foods that survive their trip through the gastrointestinal tract and feed our microbiota (community of microbes). Since probiotics aren't "digested," they have a lower caloric impact on your body, which can help you lose weight. Prebiotics are a special kind of high-fiber food that isn't digested and goes on to stimulate healthy communities of gut bugs by giving them something substantial to nibble on. And since 90 percent of our cells are actually non-human microbes, we should know how to feed them properly. Two of the most widely studied prebiotic compounds are inulin and oligofructose, and the following five foods are bursting with them:

JERUSALEM ARTICHOKES

ASPARAGUS

DANDELION GREENS

ONIONS

BANANAS

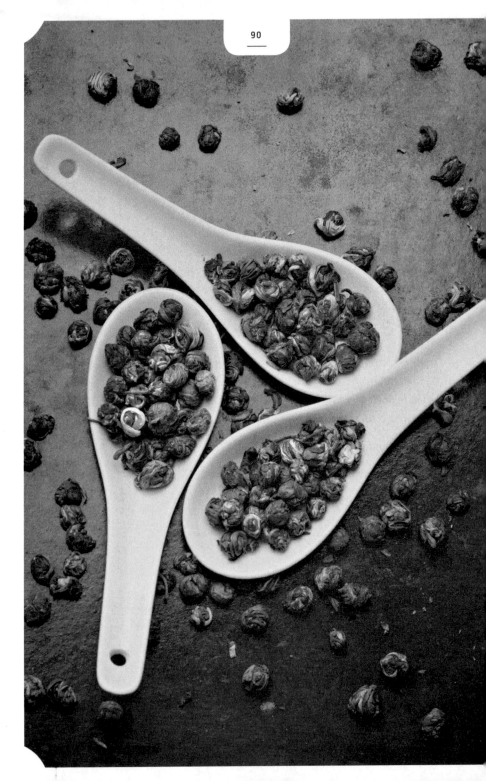

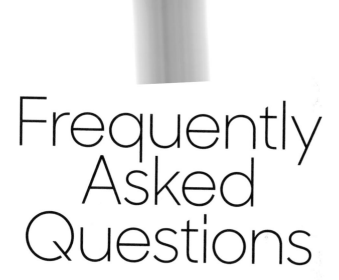

Frequently Asked Questions

All your weight-loss worries, solved!

FREQUENTLY ASKED QUESTIONS

1 What if I didn't drink the exact amount of green tea you suggest? Do I have to drink more the next day to make up for it?

No. Achieving perfection every day isn't realistic. Try to adhere as closely as possible to the principles of the *17-Day Green Tea Diet* every day, but don't be too hard on yourself if you miss a few steps. There's always tomorrow!

2 Today was a particularly stressful day, and I just couldn't resist the last box of cookies! What do I do?

Don't dwell on your binge. Everyone slips up sometimes. Next time you get a snack attack, though, reach for a cup of green tea. It not only helps quell your hunger but also boosts your metabolism, burning fat instead of storing it.

3 How long is my tea good for once I've opened it?

The most abundant green tea catechin, EGCG, has been shown to decrease 28 percent during six months of storage in homelike conditions, while the second most abundant tea catechin decreased 51 percent. Thus, it's best to drink green tea as fresh as possible to enjoy the sensory and potential health benefits of these phytochemicals. Storing tea in sealed packaging in cool, dark conditions helps increase shelf life.

While fresh may be best for enjoying many types of teas, that's not

4 What's better, tea bags or loose tea? Money's tight, and loose teas are pricey.

A report by ConsumerLab.com, an independent site that tests health products, found that green tea brewed from loose tea leaves was perhaps the best and most potent source of antioxidants like EGCG, though plain and simple tea bags made by Lipton and Bigelow were the most cost-efficient source. A single serving of Teavana's Gyokuro green tea, about a teaspoonful, was chock-full of antioxidants, yielding about 250 milligrams of catechins, a third of which were EGCG. A single bag of the green tea sold by Lipton and Bigelow contained somewhat smaller amounts of antioxidants than Teavana's green tea. But Teavana's recommended serving size was large, and the tea was also far more expensive, resulting in a higher cost per serving. The report calculated that the cost to obtain 200 milligrams of EGCG ranged from 27 cents to 60 cents with the tea bags versus $2.18 with the Teavana loose tea leaves. Tea brews made from loose tea leaves and tea bags did not differ appreciably in folic acid content, but tea bags can inhibit folic acid extraction. So while loose leaves are the best, they're both more expensive and less convenient. Save them for special moments, and rest assured that your regular tea bag is doing more than enough to help turbocharge your weight loss. And if your wallet does permit, consider matcha tea for its remarkable potency and deep, rich flavor.

5 I really don't have the time to measure the temperature of my water when I make tea.
How much will temperature affect the taste and efficacy?

Just use hot water—don't get too caught up in the exact temps. In fact, simply taking a boiling kettle off the heat and letting it sit for 30 to 60 seconds before pouring should bring it right into the perfect range. But even cold water will work in a pinch, although you may need to let the tea steep longer.

6 I've heard most tea bags use toxins and harsh bleaches to dye them nice and white. Is it true?
Is it dangerous?

Tea bags are made from a paper that is composed of wood and vegetable fibers. Oftentimes, this paper is bleached for appearance, and then the tea leaves and herbs are sealed inside using a thermoplastic material. There are a number of teas that market themselves as dioxin-, whitener-, and epichlorohydrin-free; however, in our extensive research, we couldn't find hard science or an official report that says there are any known downsides to standard tea bags. Most of the sources of this info weren't too reputable.

... in the spring of 2015 when one man fell
... from drinking massive amounts of tea, resulting in an oxalate
intake of 1,500 milligrams per day. (He was drinking 16 large iced
teas a day!) The Academy of Nutrition and Dietetics advises consuming no more than 40 to 50 milligrams of oxalate per day.

But even that number is hard to reach. While the amount of oxalate you receive from a cup of tea varies depending on the amount of
tea in the bag and the steeping time, only black tea has significant
levels of oxalate—and even then, you'd need to drink a lot of it to even
approach hazardous levels. Here's how much oxalate you'll find in a
typical cup of tea:

- Black tea: 1.36–12.6mg/cup
- Green tea: 0.23–4.36mg/cup
- White tea: 0.40–3.6mg/cup
- Oolong tea: 0.23–6mg/cup
- Herbal tea: In general, herbal teas have indetectable amounts of oxalate. Most go up to about 0.6mg per cup, max
- Rooibos: Indetectable amounts

So while you'll be drinking about five cups of green tea a day on this
diet (including the smoothies), they do not have significant levels of
oxalate.

8 How do I store my teas? And how long are they really good for unopened?

EGCG, the active ingredient in green tea, is highly unstable under sunlight. Keep tea in a dark, dry place. Storing tea in sealed packaging in cool, dark conditions helps increase shelf life. If you brew iced tea, it will stay good for about four days, as long as you keep it refrigerated. The long-term stability of green tea catechins like EGCG in canned and bottled drinks is currently unknown. What we do know is that store-bought bottled teas typically lose 20 percent of EGCG/catechin content during the bottling process. If you really want bottled tea, then shoot for versions with an acid like lemon juice or citric acid, which helps stabilize EGCG levels.

9 My iced tea seems to get cloudy after I brew it. Does that mean it's gone bad?

Not at all. The natural oil in the brewed tea will create cloudiness if you haven't cooled it to room temperature before refrigerating. Though it may not be very attractive, it's still fine to drink. If you've refrigerated tea too soon, and it has that slightly opaque look, just pour in some boiling water (1 cup per quart of iced tea) and stir to clear it. Clouding is typically caused by the precipitation of the tannins in the tea. Stronger teas and more high-quality teas cloud faster because they have higher levels of tannins. Clouding can also be caused by minerals in your water, which are harmless. But if the effect bothers you, you may want to use a water filter.

...........ιΓαΙΥ larger waists and chances of being obese than those in the lowest quartile.

11 How is decaffeinated tea made? Is it harmful?

There are a number of ways tea may be decaffeinated. Up until the mid-1970s, all decaffeination was performed using organic solvents, but then concerns about the side effects of solvents on both the body and the environment led the industry to find alternative methods. Here are the more common ones:

Ethyl acetate: One of the most common methods now used involves ethyl acetate, also known as acetic acid ethyl ester. Ethyl acetate is an ester and is a clear, volatile, and flammable liquid, with a fruity flavor and a pleasant taste when diluted. Because it is found in many fruits, such as apples, peaches, and pears, and is completely digestible, it has been used in a wide range of foods, such as salad dressings and fruit desserts, and has been approved for decaffeination by the FDA since 1982.

Carbon dioxide: This is an ideal method with no toxic residues, less degradation of the tea catechins, and a high retention of the tea flavors. However, it's expensive to set up and not used as widely as it could be.

Water: Water decaffeination is done by first blanching freshly harvested green tea leaves in boiling water for a short period of time. Because the water solubility of caffeine is higher than the solubility of the tea catechins, most of the caffeine can quickly be extracted into the boiling water, whereas the catechins mostly remain behind in the tea leaves. The leaves are then quickly removed from the boiling water, which now contains the caffeine, and are then dried to obtain decaffeinated dried green tea.

12 I feel like I get jittery drinking all this tea. What should I do? I've lost a few pounds, and I don't want to stop this diet.

Try to incorporate some decaf varieties. Many people avoid decaffeinated tea, believing that its beneficial properties are lost in the decaffeination process. However, the effect on polyphenols (the antioxidants) is considered to be marginal.

13 What is Fair Trade tea?

Fair Trade Certified tea comes from both cooperatives and from large farms. Fair Trade helps tea farmers and workers gain access to capital, set fair prices for their products, and make democratic decisions about how to best improve their businesses, their communities, and their tea. Fair Trade certification protects tea estate workers as it ensures fair labor conditions and fair minimum wages. Fair Trade farmers gain access to international markets and are empowered to build organizational capacity to compete in the global marketplace. A minimum sales price is guaranteed to ensure a sustainable wage is paid to tea workers and a sustainable income is paid to

one cup? After two?

A good tea will provide at least three infusions, but most of the important substances are extracted during the first infusion. So for maximum nutrient benefit, start with a fresh tea bag for each new cup. However, if you are reusing a tea bag, you can boost antioxidant levels by adding a splash of vitamin C–rich juice such as lemon, orange, or pineapple to your cup. Studies on green tea showed that these juices help you absorb 13 times the amount of antioxidants.

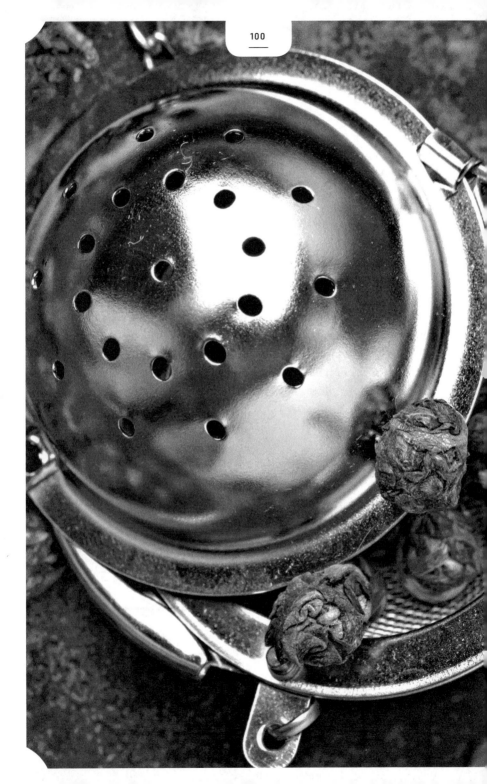

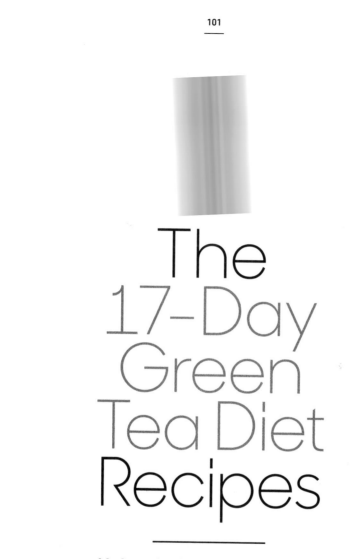

The 17-Day Green Tea Diet Recipes

Unleash the power of the Five Green Superfoods

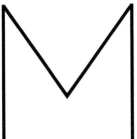ost food trends don't pass the nutritional sniff test—hot-dog-crusted pizza, anyone? But over the past few years, you've probably noticed green tea showing up in everything from lattes to cookies to energy drinks. And that's one trend we can get behind.

Although characterizing a practice that's centuries old as a "trend" might be a little narrow-minded. The Chinese have been smoking ducks and cooking eggs in tea for hundreds of years; we're only now getting hip to the idea.

In this chapter, you'll discover a number of recipes that incorporate green tea, as well as others that use the Green Superfoods in ways that help boost your levels of EGCG. But maximizing your green tea consumption doesn't have to begin and end with the ideas on these pages. Here are some time-honored ways to get more green tea into your day:

steep tea bags in oils and vinegars to create richly flavored salad dressings.

- Add powdered tea to doughs or batters—it's great in everything from cakes and cookies to pancakes and muffins.

- Chop green tea and mix it with salt and pepper for a smoky, high-potency rub.

- Use it in place of broths for soup recipes.

- Use tea as a poaching or braising liquid.

- Mix powdered tea into ice creams or whipped cream for a nutritional dessert.

And of course, your daily Green Tea Smoothie is a great opportunity to fiddle with a wide range of flavors.

Your Green Tea Smoothie Guide

Unless you've been living in an igloo for the past two decades, you should know by now that Americans do not eat enough fruits and vegetables. In fact, recent surveys have found that only about 30 percent of Americans are eating the recommended five or more servings of fruits and vegetables a day. That's a pretty pitiful performance and no doubt a partial cause of the obesity epidemic that grips this nation.

If you happen to be one of those seven out of 10 of us who don't eat enough plant matter, then you need to make fast friends with the smoothie. It's the quickest, most delicious way to make up for the fruit-and-vegetable deficit: Roll out of bed, toss some fruit in a blender, top with a bit of liquid, hit "liquefy." Boom! You're on the path to a skinnier, healthier existence.

Making smoothies can be a pretty freewheeling endeavor, which is certainly part of the fun, but we've established a few basic rules. Follow these and the ingredient-by-ingredient guide that follows and you'll be ready for liquid liftoff.

chapter uses the life-giving drink as a jumping-off point. Make a big pot of it and keep it chilling in your fridge for daily smoothie building.

RULE 2
ADD DAIRY.

We suggest ½ cup plain nonfat Greek-style yogurt. (This will ensure that there is always adequate protein.) For a thinner smoothie, you can use 2 percent milk.

RULE 3
MAKE SURE YOU HAVE FIBER.

To slow digestion, keep you full, and ensure you're hitting your daily fiber content, consider adding a fiber booster like psyllium husk or flax meal.

RULE 4
BRING ON THE FRUIT.

Adequate vitamin C is critical for maximizing your absorption of EGCG. A daily smoothie helps ensure you're up to snuff on your C intake. Your best weapon may be frozen fruit: Not only is it considerably more affordable, but research has found that frozen fruits may actually carry higher levels of antioxidants because they're picked at the height of the season and flash-frozen on the spot. Also, frozen fruit means you can use less ice to make your smoothie sufficiently cold, which in turn yields a more intense, pure flavor. (Make sure the fruit is unsweetened!)

RULE 5
USE A STRONG BLENDER.

A weak blender won't be able to crush the ice quickly enough, which means it will melt and ultimately dilute your precious creation rather than giving it that bracing, velvety texture you want.

RULE 6
RESPECT THE RATIO.

Once you learn the basic proportions of liquids to solids, you can turn anything into a pretty drinkable smoothie. For every 3 cups of fruit, you'll need about 1 cup of tea. Keep in mind that both yogurt and ice will thicken your drink.

. . . . (1 cup)

107 calories / 24g sugars / 3g fiber

This tropical treasure has become increasingly available in American supermarkets in both fresh and frozen forms. Yes, it's higher in sugar than almost any other fruit in the produce section, but it also brings to the blender three-quarters of your day's vitamin C and 25 percent of your vitamin A. Consider added sweeteners entirely superfluous when making smoothies with mango.

PAPAYA *(1 cup)*
55 calories / 8g sugars / 3g fiber

Is there any fruit better for you than papaya? Flooded with vitamin C, replete with vision-strengthening vitamin A, and blessed with one of the most favorable fiber-to-sugar ratios imaginable, papaya proves itself to be one of the most well-rounded foods on the planet. Papaya also boasts papain and chymopapain, two potent enzymes that have been shown to fight inflammation, the cause of asthma, arthritis, and other serious conditions.

KIWI *(1 fruit)*
54 calories / 8g sugars / 2.5g fiber

A half-cup of kiwi—a berry that originated in China, despite its iden-tification with New Zealand—gives you almost 150 percent of your daily vitamin C and is also a good source of vitamin K, potassium, and omega-3 fatty acids. But the unique power of the kiwi may stem from its uniquely green flesh, the result of its high levels of chlorophyll, which helps our bodies grow and repair tissue and improve oxygen flow throughout the body.

STRAWBERRIES *(1 cup)*
49 calories / 7g sugars / 3g fiber

Beyond the monster dose of vitamin C (calorie for calorie, you'll get more C than you'd find in an orange), strawberries also prove to be a rich source of phenols, including the same brain-boosting, anti-inflammatory anthocyanins found in blueberries. They also lay claim to a rare and powerful antioxidant called ellagitannin, which has been shown to provide a stout defense against a variety of cancers.

BANANA *(1 medium)*
105 calories / 14g sugars / 3g fiber

Sure, there are fruits with deeper nutritional portfolios, but the humble banana serves as an all-star utility player in the smoothie game. Not only does it offer a handful of hard-to-find nutrients (heart-strengthening potassium, gut-friendly prebiotics), but it also provides smoothies with a balanced, creamy texture and enough natural sweetness to ensure no need for added sugar. Peel a few very ripe bananas, stick them in a plastic bag, and toss them in the freezer. (Make sure you peel them before you freeze them, because the ice box turns their skins into little yellow Kevlar vests.)

... impressive fiber load and you have the makings of a seriously satisfying smoothie. Plus, avocados add a richness that makes it feel like you're splurging, even when you're not.

PINEAPPLE *(1 cup)*
82 calories / 16g sugars / 2g fiber

Feeling low on energy? A cup of pineapple might just be the antidote. That's because pineapple is one of nature's best sources of manganese, a trace mineral that is essential for energy production. A cup provides 76 percent of your daily recommended intake, making pineapple nature's answer to Red Bull.

PEACH *(1 fruit)*
60 calories / 13 g sugars / 2 g fiber

Peaches pack lutein and zeaxanthin, powerful carotenoids proven to help protect your peepers from macular degeneration. Plus, the blast of beta carotene may help stave off heart disease and cancer. But a USDA survey found that peaches are the most pesticide-laden fruit in the produce section, so if you can afford organic, you might want to spring.

THICKENERS & ENHANCERS

PEANUT BUTTER *(1 tablespoon)*
94 calories / 8g fat (1.5g saturated) / 1g sugars / 3.5g protein

What's not to love about peanut butter? The fat is good for your heart, the protein is good for your muscles, and the package of vitamins and nutrients (vitamin E, manganese, niacin) will do plenty for the rest of your body. The only drawback is that peanut butter is extremely dense with calories (and don't bother with the reduced-fat stuff—it's loaded with chemicals), so try to keep the quantity to about half a tablespoon per smoothie.

GREEK-STYLE YOGURT *(½ cup)*
70 calories / 0g fat / 5g sugars / 12g protein

There may be no better addition to a smoothie than a healthy scoop of Greek yogurt. Not only does it give the smoothie a lovely body, but it also adds a ton of protein and gut-friendly bacteria to whatever concoction it graces. Why Greek? Because the Greeks are savvy enough to skim off the watery whey found in typical yogurt, thus yielding a creamier product with more than twice the protein found in the Dannons and the Yoplaits of the dairy world. Both Fage and Oikos are reliable brands found in most supermarkets. If you must stick to regular American-style yogurt, just make sure it's unflavored; opt for a fruit- or vanilla-flavored yogurt and you might as well be using ice cream.

....., ...u sugar in any form is highly discouraged in the craft of smoothie making, so use honey sparingly, if at all.

FRESH MINT/FRESH BASIL *(2 tablespoons)*
2 calories / 0g fa / 0g sugars

Strange though it may sound, adding fresh herbs to smoothies is a small little trick that yields big results when properly employed. Plus, when you consider that fresh basil contains cancer-fighting carotenoids and that the menthol in mint can help facilitate easy breathing and relieve indigestion, what more motivation do you need? Basil pairs well with strawberries and watermelon, while mint works wonders on melon, blueberries, and papaya.

AGAVE SYRUP *(1 tablespoon)*
60 calories / 0g fat / 15g sugars

Let's be clear: As long as your smoothie is composed primarily of fruit, there is no reason to add sugar to the mix. But if you ever do reach for it, agave syrup is the way to go. The sweetness comes primarily from a form of fructose called inulin, which has a very gentle effect on your blood sugar. This not only helps prevent the dreaded sugar crash but also keeps your body from going into fat-storage mode. Score a bottle at most health-food stores and grocers like Whole Foods.

BOOSTS

PROTEIN POWDER *(2 tablespoons)*
104 calories / 0g fat / 16g protein

No, protein powder isn't just for the muscle-mag set. Dozens of studies have highlighted the importance of getting protein first thing in the morning. Not only will it help jolt your metabolism into action, but it's also been shown to help you retain focus throughout the morning.

FIBER POWDER *(2 tablespoons)*
35 calories / 0g fat / 3–6g fiber

Often sold under the name "psyllium husk" (for the seeds this powder is ground from), a dose of fiber is going to do more than promote a healthy colon. Fiber will slow the digestion of the smoothie in your stomach, which means not only will you stay fuller longer but also the sugar from the fruit will have a less dramatic impact on your blood sugar levels. And if the Quaker Oats dude has taught us anything, it's that fiber promotes a healthy heart as well.

FISH OIL *(1 teaspoon)*
41 calories / 5g fat (1g saturated) / 1,084mg omega-3s

Fish oil has been canonized by hordes of wide-eyed nutritionists over the years, and the case for its sainthood sure is compelling. The tide of omega-3 fatty acids found in fish oil (usually made from fatty fish

GROUND FLAXSEED *(2 tablespoons)*
80 calories / 5g fat (1g saturated) / 2,700mg omega-3s

These seeds, picked and ground from the flax plant commonly found across the Mediterranean and Middle East, deliver a mother lode of omega-3s. Consider stirring them into your oatmeal or yogurt, but if you're looking for the easiest way to sneak flax into your diet, use the blender for seamless integration.

WHEATGRASS POWDER *(1.25 tablespoons)*
35 calories

What doesn't wheatgrass offer? Even a tiny dose like this packs fiber, protein, tons of vitamin A and K, folic acid, manganese, iodine, and chlrophyll, to name a few. You don't need to know what each nutrient does for you; just know that a single tablespoon will have you operating at peak performance levels. Pick some up at AmazingGrass.com.

Smoothie Recipes

The Green Banana

1 ripe banana

½ cup green tea

½ cup 2 percent milk

1 tablespoon peanut butter

1 tablespoon agave syrup

1 cup ice

With protein, healthy fat, and caffeine, this works perfectly as a start to your day or as a low-cal substitute for a milk shake.

311 calories / 52g carbs / 10g protein / 4g fiber

The Purple Monster

1 cup blueberries

½ cup strawberries

½ cup green tea

½ cup fat-free Greek-style yogurt

3 or 4 ice cubes

1 tablespoon flaxseed

Between the polyphenols in the blueberries and strawberries and the omega-3s in the flax, we're talking serious brain food.

248 calories / 42g carbs / 16g protein / 9g fiber

¾ cup frozen mango

½ cup carrot juice

½ cup green tea

½ cup fat-free Greek-style yogurt

1 tablespoon protein powder

½ cup water

All that orange produce means this baby is stuffed full of vision-strengthening, cancer-fighting carotenoids.

218 calories / 42g carbs / 13g protein / 7g fiber

The Papaya Berry

¾ cup frozen papaya

¾ cup frozen strawberries

½ cup 2 percent milk

½ cup green tea

1 tablespoon fresh mint

This is like a liquid multivitamin, loaded with vitamins A and C, plus disease-fighting carotenoids and lycopene.

250 calories / 52g carbs / 16g protein / 5g fiber

The Pineapple Punch

1 cup frozen pineapple

½ cup Greek-style yogurt

½ cup 2 percent milk

½ cup green tea

Like a tropical island in a glass. In fact, a shot of rum would turn this into one heck of a healthy cocktail.

215 calories / 37g carbs / 18g protein / 4g fiber

The Green Goddess

¼ avocado, peeled and pitted

1 ripe banana

1 tablespoon honey

½ cup green tea

1 scoop protein powder

½ cup ice

Optional: 1 teaspoon freshly grated ginger

Fiber and protein combine forces to vanquish any hunger in this untraditional but tasty creation.

300 calories / 50g carbs / 18g protein / 6g fiber

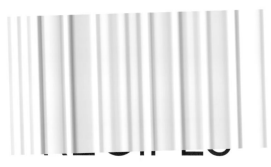

The power of green tea is such that it has been shown to strip away pounds even while you go about your regular diet! In fact, a 2015 study in the journal *Food & Function* found that green tea reduced body weight, fat accumulation, inflammation, and even levels of leptin—the "hunger hormone"—in animals fed a high-fat diet.

But when you have such a potent weapon at your disposal, why not use it to its maximum capacity? The *17-Day Green Tea Diet* is a weight-loss Maserati. Don't keep it in the garage! These recipes will help you open up the engine and send your fat burners into the red.

LUNCH
Matcha Salad
Green Superfoods

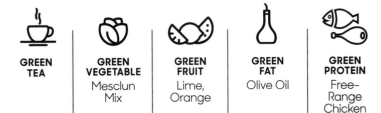

GREEN TEA	GREEN VEGETABLE	GREEN FRUIT	GREEN FAT	GREEN PROTEIN
	Mesclun Mix	Lime, Orange	Olive Oil	Free-Range Chicken

This simple salad uses powdered green tea to create a smoky, savory dressing, while the orange brings out the power of the EGCG in the matcha and the folate in the greens.

FOR THE DRESSING

1 teaspoon matcha green tea powder

1 tablespoon olive oil

1 tablespoon lime juice

Dash of salt and pepper

FOR THE SALAD

1 cup chopped mesclun mix

½ red onion, thinly sliced

2 large red radishes, thinly sliced

1 large orange, broken into sections

1 small free-range chicken breast, grilled and cut into chunks

MAKES 1 SERVINGS

406 cal / 17 g fat (2 g saturated) / 433 mg sodium

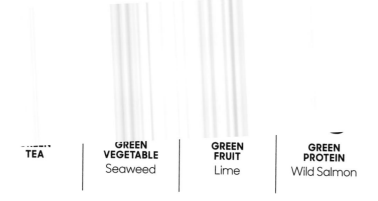

TEA	GREEN VEGETABLE	GREEN FRUIT	GREEN PROTEIN
	Seaweed	Lime	Wild Salmon

Ochazuke is a quickie foodie trick from Japan. It's made by pouring a cup of hot green tea over a bowl of rice, then topping the bowl with savory ingredients. We've made this dish particularly *17-Day Green Tea Diet*–friendly.

1 cup cooked or leftover white rice

1 cup green tea

3 rice crackers, broken into small pieces

1 cup flaked wild salmon (leftover, or from a packet)

½ cup dried seaweed

Juice of ½ lime

Low-sodium soy sauce

→ Place the rice in a bowl. Pour the hot tea over it. Top with crackers, salmon, seaweed, lime juice, and soy sauce.

MAKES 3 SERVINGS

409 cal / 1.7 g fat (0 g saturated) / 1,144 mg sodium

Matcha Scrambled Eggs

Green Superfoods

GREEN TEA

GREEN VEGETABLE
Asparagus

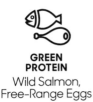

GREEN PROTEIN
Wild Salmon,
Free-Range Eggs

Two eggs scrambled in a pat of butter contain approximately 200 calories. So how does Denny's get from 200 to 1,150 with their Heartland Scramble? And how do so many other restaurants sling together scrambles with more than 1,000 calories? Simple: excessive oil and egregious amounts of cheese. This scramble has all the makings of hearty breakfast fare—butter, cheese, protein—but with healthy fats, fresh vegetables, and a light caloric toll. Serve it with a scoop of roasted potatoes and fresh fruit.

1	Tbsp butter
8	stalks asparagus, woody bottoms removed, chopped into 1" pieces
	Salt and black pepper to taste
8	eggs
2	Tbsp fat-free milk
¼	cup crumbled fresh goat cheese
4	oz smoked salmon, chopped
1	Tbsp matcha powder

, ... and scrape the eggs until they begin to form soft curds. A minute before they're done, stir in the goat cheese.

→ Remove from the heat when the eggs are still creamy and soft (remember, scrambled eggs are like meat—they continue to cook even after you cut the heat) and fold in the smoked salmon.

→ Mix 1 teaspoon of matcha with coarse sea salt and black pepper. Sprinkle over eggs.

MAKES 4 SERVINGS

320 calories / 17 g fat (6 g saturated) / 540 mg sodium

Tuna Snack Wraps with Strawberry Salad

Green Superfoods

GREEN VEGETABLE
Spinach

GREEN FRUIT
Strawberries

GREEN FAT
Avocado, Walnuts

GREEN PROTEIN
Tuna, Free-Range Eggs

TUNA WRAPS

1	lb canned light chunk tuna, drained
¼	cup mayonnaise
½	avocado, diced
2	hard-boiled eggs, diced
½	medium red onion, sliced thin
	Salt and pepper
12	bibb lettuce leaves (about 1 head)

SALAD

2	cups packed baby spinach
1	cup strawberries, quartered
2	tbsp vinaigrette dressing
2	tbsp raw walnuts, toasted in a dry pan over medium heat until fragrant (about 2 minutes), and roughly chopped

→ Combine all the salad ingredients in a bowl and mix well.

→ Divide the salad among four plates. Serve with three lettuce wraps.

MAKES 4 SERVINGS

304 calories / 15 g fat / 9 g carb / 6 g fiber / 24 g protein

Wahoo Tacos

Green Superfoods

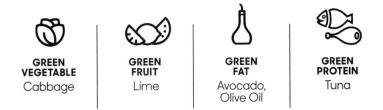

GREEN VEGETABLE	**GREEN FRUIT**	**GREEN FAT**	**GREEN PROTEIN**
Cabbage	Lime	Avocado, Olive Oil	Tuna

Taco night in the average American home generally means ground beef, crunchy shells, and shredded cheese. Nothing wrong with that, but other meat and fish can deliver more flavor for a fraction of the calories. Exhibit A: ahi tuna. Not only does the combination of silky rare tuna and creamy avocado fit a boatload of healthy fat into the palm of your hand, but the flavors are tough to beat, especially when crowned with a spicy slaw and the tang of a few pickled onions. Forget the fried version: This is your new fish taco.

4	cups shredded red or green cabbage
2	Tbsp olive oil mayonnaise
	Juice of 1 lime, plus lime wedges for serving
½	Tbsp canned chipotle pepper
	Salt and black pepper to taste
½	Tbsp canola or olive oil
12	oz fresh ahi or other high-quality tuna
8	corn tortillas
1	ripe avocado, pitted, peeled, and sliced
	Pickled Red Onion
	Hot sauce

2 minutes on each side, until a nice crust has developed but the inside of the tuna is still rare.

→ While the pan is still hot, heat the tortillas until lightly crisp on the outside.

→ Slice the tuna into thin planks. Divide among the tortillas and top each with avocado slices, slaw, and pickled onions. Serve with lime wedges and hot sauce.

MAKES 4 SERVINGS

330 calories / 13 g fat (2 g saturated) / 460 mg sodium

Crabacado Salad

Green Superfoods

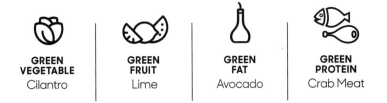

GREEN VEGETABLE	**GREEN FRUIT**	**GREEN FAT**	**GREEN PROTEIN**
Cilantro	Lime	Avocado	Crab Meat

Crab doesn't come out much in the kitchen, but when it does, the idea is to do as little to it as possible. Otherwise, why spend the money on such a delicate ingredient? With the exception of a few salty Marylanders, nobody knows crabs better than the cooks of Southeast Asia, so we follow their light-handed lead here. Cucumber and onion for crunch, chiles for heat, and a bit of fish or soy sauce for a slick of savory salt. An avocado half makes the perfect vessel for this salad, its rich, creamy texture boosting the sweetness of the crab.

1	can (8 oz) crabmeat, preferably jumbo lump, drained
½	cup diced seeded and peeled cucumber
¼	cup minced red onion
¼	cup chopped cilantro
1	jalapeño pepper (preferably red), minced
1	Tbsp fish sauce (in a pinch, soy sauce will do)
1	Tbsp sugar
	Juice of 1 lime
	Salt
4	small Hass avocados, halved and pitted
1	lime, quartered

THE 17-DAY GREEN TEA DIET

MAKES 4 SERVINGS

355 calories / 25 g fat (4 g saturated) / 550 mg sodium

Star of Noodle Soup

Green Superfoods

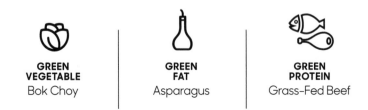

**GREEN
VEGETABLE**
Bok Choy

**GREEN
FAT**
Asparagus

**GREEN
PROTEIN**
Grass-Fed Beef

When it comes to soups that serve as meals, no one can touch the Asian cuisines. From the thick, heady ramens of Japan to the funky, darkly satisfying beef noodle soups of China, to the spice-suffused bowls of pho from Vietnam, the entire continent seems to have mastered the art of transforming a few scraps of meat and vegetables into a magical eating experience. The slow-cooker soup here takes a cue from all three, combining a rich ginger- and soy-spiked broth with chunks of fork-tender beef, a tangle of springy noodles, and—for a fresh, high note to pair with the dark, brooding ones—a pile of fresh bok choy. This is no appetizer soup; this is a full-on meal.

½ Tbsp peanut or canola oil

1½ pounds grass-fed chuck roast, cut into ½" chunks

Salt and black pepper to taste

4 cups low-sodium beef stock

6 cups water

¼ cup low-sodium soy sauce

2 medium onions, roughly chopped

4 cloves garlic, peeled

1" piece peeled fresh ginger, sliced into thin coins

4 whole star anise pods

the beef on all sides for 3 to 4 minutes, until browned. Transfer to a slow cooker and add the stock, water, soy sauce, onions, garlic, ginger, and star anise. Cook on low for 6 hours, until the beef is very tender. (Or, simmer everything in the pot over a very low flame for 2 to 3 hours.)

→ When the beef is nearly ready, prepare the noodles according to package instructions. Add the bok choy to the soup and simmer for about 10 minutes, until tender. Season to taste with salt (if it needs any) and plenty of black pepper. Divide the noodles among 8 large bowls. Ladle the broth, along with a generous amount of beef and bok choy, into each bowl. Top with any of the garnishes you like.

MAKES 8 SERVINGS

350 calories / 8 g fat (2 g saturated) / 550 mg sodium

Seize Your Salad

Green Superfoods

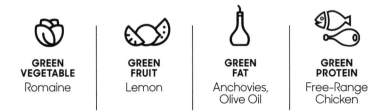

GREEN VEGETABLE	GREEN FRUIT	GREEN FAT	GREEN PROTEIN
Romaine	Lemon	Anchovies, Olive Oil	Free-Range Chicken

Caesar salad may be the most misleading food in America—it's the type of dish you order when you want to be good to your body, only to find out it's eating up half of your day's calories. This recipe transforms the high-calorie dressing into a lighter vinaigrette and adds substance, flavor, and nutrition in the form of sundried tomatoes and olives.

DRESSING

- 2 Tbsp red wine vinegar
- 1 Tbsp mayonnaise
- 1 clove garlic, minced
- 2 anchovies (soak in milk for 10 minutes if you want to mellow the flavor)
- 1 tsp Worcestershire sauce

  Juice of 1 lemon
- 6–8 turns of a black-pepper mill
- ½ cup olive oil

SALAD

- 4 hearts of romaine
- 2 English muffins, split

THE 17-DAY GREEN TEA DIET

→ Preheat the grill. Combine all the dressing ingredients except the oil in a food processor and pulse to blend. With the motor running, slowly drizzle in the oil.

→ Cut the romaine down the middle lengthwise, leaving the root end intact so the leaves hold together. Brush the romaine, English muffins, and chicken with olive oil and season with salt and pepper. When the grill is hot, add the chicken and grill for 4 to 5 minutes per side until firm and caramelized. Remove the chicken and allow to rest.

→ Place the lettuce and English muffins on the grill. Cook the lettuce for 1 to 2 minutes, just enough to lightly char and wilt the leaves. Cook the English muffins until brown and crispy.

→ Slice the chicken into thin strips. Cut the muffins into bite-size pieces. Arrange both, along with the olives and sundried tomatoes, over the individual lettuce halves. Drizzle with dressing and sprinkle with cheese.

MAKES 4 SERVINGS

410 calories / 29 g fat (3.5 g saturated) / 610 mg sodium

THE *17-DAY GREEN TEA DIET* RECIPES

DINNER

Green-Tea-Poached Wild Salmon with Bok Choy

Green Superfoods

			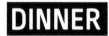
GREEN TEA	**GREEN FRUIT** Bok Choy	**GREEN FAT** Lime, Orange	**GREEN PROTEIN** Wild Salmon

POACHING LIQUID

- 2 qts water
- 5 tbsp loose green tea, or 5 green tea bags
- 2 inch piece fresh ginger, peeled and sliced thin
- 3 tbsp reduced sodium tamari
- Juice of 2 limes
- Zest of 1 orange
- 4 tbsp raw Manuka honey
- Salt and pepper to taste

- 4 5 oz portions of wild salmon
- 2 tbsp extra virgin olive oil
- 1 lb bok choy, cored and sliced lengthwise
- 1 Tbsp water

→ While the poaching liquid simmers, season the fish with salt and pepper and set aside.

→ Once the broth has simmered for 10 minutes, turn of the heat. Season the liquid with salt and fresh black pepper to taste; it should be very flavorful.

→ Place the the salmon in the pot and leave to poach in the hot liquid, off the heat, for about 7 to 8 minutes.

→ While the salmon is poaching, heat a large sauté pan over medium heat. Add the olive oil and the bok choy to the pan. Add a tablespoon of water to the pan to help the leafy green steam.

→ Add the sofrito to the pan. Cook the bok choy until tender— about 4 to 5 minutes total, turning every one or town minutes.

→ Divide the bok choy among four plates. Use a slotted spoon to carefully lift the salmon out of the poaching liquid. Place on top of the bok choy. Squeeze the juice of one orange on top of all four fillets. Serve immediately.

MAKES 4 SERVINGS

413 calories / 16 g fat / 34 g carb / 4 g fiber / 34 g protein

*To make sofrito, combine 1 seeded serrano chili, ⅓ cup coarsely chopped shallots, ⅓ cup coarsely chopped ginger, and ½ cup extra-virgin olive oil in a saucepan and wok over low heat until shallots are very soft, about 8 minutes.

Chicken & Chard

Green Superfoods

**GREEN
VEGETABLE**
Swiss Chard,
Basil

**GREEN
FRUIT**
Lemon

**GREEN
FAT**
Olive Oil

**GREEN
PROTEIN**
Free-Range
Chicken

4	5 oz boneless skinless chicken breasts
	Salt and pepper
2	cups Zero Belly Marinara or storebought
½	lb swiss chard, rinsed of dirt and patted dry
1	tbsp extra virgin olive oil
¼	cup water
½	lemon
½	cup roughly choppedfresh basil (optional)
2	cups cooked brown rice
	Olive oil spray

→ Preheat the oven to 350°F.

→ Heat a nonstick pan, lightly coated with olive oil spray over medium heat.

→ Season the chicken breast with a pinch of salt and pepper, and sear in the pan until lightly golden brown, about 3 minutes on each side. Don't worry about cooking the chicken breast all the way through. Place the seared chicken in a glass casserole dish.

→ Pour the marinara over the chicken breast and cover the dish with foil. Place in the oven and cook for 15 minutes.

→ While the chicken cooks, prepare the swiss chard. Take the green leaves of the stems and roughly chop. Thinly slice the

Top with one chicken breast and marinara. Serve with ½ cup brown rice. Garnish with basil.

MAKES 4 SERVINGS

300 calories / 3 g fat / 38 g carbs / 6 g fiber / 39 g protein

Scallops Chimichurri in a Hurry

Green Superfoods

GREEN VEGETABLE	**GREEN FAT**	**GREEN PROTEIN**
Parsley	Olive Oil	Scallops

Chimichurri is an herb-based sauce from Argentina used to adorn and enhance a variety of different dishes, grilled meats and fish above all. After some careful reflection, we've decided that chimi is pretty much the world's greatest condiment, turning bad food good and making good food great. Once you make it, you'll have a hard time not painting it on everything you come across: sandwiches, grilled vegetables, eggs. So it's probably worthwhile to double the recipe and have a bit stashed in the fridge for when cravings strike, which will be often after you make this dish.

½ cup water

　　Salt

2　Tbsp red wine vinegar

1　cup fresh parsley, chopped

2　cloves garlic, minced

　　Pinch red pepper flakes

3　Tbsp olive oil

1　lb large sea scallops

　　Black pepper to taste

➙ Heat the remaining 1 tablespoon oil in a large skillet over medium-high heat. Thoroughly dry the scallops with paper towels, then season on both sides with salt and pepper. When the oil is hot, add the scallops and cook for 2 to 3 minutes on the first side, without disturbing them, until a deep brown crust has developed. Flip and cook for 1 to 2 minutes longer, until firm but yielding to the touch. Serve drizzled with the chimichurri.

MAKES 4 SERVINGS

200 calories / 11 g fat (1.5 g saturated) / 480 mg sodium

Alamo Steak Salad

Green Superfoods

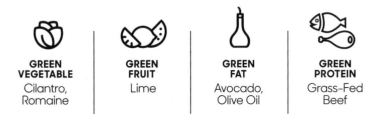

GREEN VEGETABLE	GREEN FRUIT	GREEN FAT	GREEN PROTEIN
Cilantro, Romaine	Lime	Avocado, Olive Oil	Grass-Fed Beef

We've long lamented the Mexican-style restaurant salad, in all of its greasy, overwrought, hypercaloric absurdity. Whether from the drive-thru or at a sit-down establishment, no salad is likely to be worse for you than the one with "fiesta" or "olé" or "Southwest" in the title. That's too bad, because the flavors that define the cuisine of our neighbors to the south should form the perfect base for an intensely satisfying, relatively healthy lunch or dinner. We've reengineered the standard, underachieving Mexican salad to be just that.

3   corn tortillas, cut into thin strips

4   small Roma tomatoes, chopped

1   red onion, diced

1   jalapeño pepper, minced

½   cup chopped fresh cilantro

J   uice of 1 lime

8   oz flank steak

    Salt and black pepper to taste

½   Tbsp red wine vinegar

1   tsp canned chipotle pepper

½   Tbsp honey

2   Tbsp olive oil

1 head

...atoes, onion, jalapeño, cilantro, and half the lime juice. Set the salsa aside.

→ Preheat a grill or grill pan. Season the steak with salt and pepper. Once the grill or pan is fully heated, toss on the steak. Cook for 4 to 5 minutes per side, depending on thickness, until firm but yielding. Let the steak rest for 5 minutes before slicing it thinly against the grain of the meat.

→ Combine the remaining lime juice with the vinegar, chipotle, and honey. Slowly drizzle in the olive oil, whisking to combine. Toss the lettuce with enough vinaigrette to lightly coat, then divide among 4 plates. Top each serving with slices of steak, black beans, avocado, a heaping spoonful of salsa, and a few tortilla strips.

MAKES 4 SERVINGS

340 calories / 18 g fat (4 g saturated) / 460 mg sodium

Chicken Fried Green Tea Rice

Green Superfoods

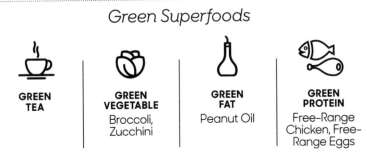

GREEN TEA	GREEN VEGETABLE	GREEN FAT	GREEN PROTEIN
	Broccoli, Zucchini	Peanut Oil	Free-Range Chicken, Free-Range Eggs

The name says it all: One of the most nutritionally dubious staples (white rice) combined with the most treacherous technique (frying). The calorie counts are predictably strato-spheric; even a small scoop used as a base for a stir-fry will run around 500 calories. More important, it contains little to no true nutrition. Our recipe turns fried rice on its head, relying on a ton of fresh produce, considerably less rice, and a bit of oil for crisping it up.

- 2 cups water
- 4 green tea bags
- 4 cups brown rice
- 1 Tbsp peanut or vegetable oil
- 4 scallions, greens and whites separated, chopped
- 1 Tbsp grated fresh ginger
- 2 cloves garlic, minced
- 1 medium zucchini, diced
- 2 carrots, diced
- 2 cups bite-size broccoli florets
- 2 cups mushrooms (preferably shiitake), stems removed, sliced

½   lb boneless

. rice has

water, about 20 minutes.

→ In a wok or a large nonstick skillet, heat the oil over medium-high heat. When the oil is lightly smoking, add the scallion whites, ginger, and garlic and cook for 30 to 45 seconds. Add the zucchini, carrots, broccoli, and mushrooms and cook for 4 to 5 minutes, using a spatula to stir the vegetables throughout. Add the chicken and continue cooking for 2 to 3 minutes, until the pieces are no longer pink.

→ Stir in the rice and soy sauce and cook for another 5 minutes, allowing the rice to get crispy on the bottom. Create an empty space in the middle of the pan and add the eggs. Use a spoon or the spatula to quickly scramble the eggs until light and fluffy, then stir them into the rest of the ingredients. Serve garnished with the scallion greens.

MAKES 4 SERVINGS

390 calories / 10 g fat (2.5 g saturated) / 720 mg sodium

Miso Tofu Bowls

Green Superfoods

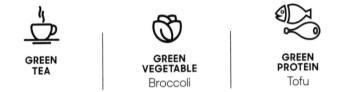

| **GREEN TEA** | **GREEN VEGETABLE** Broccoli | **GREEN PROTEIN** Tofu |

Sometimes the best way to approach cooking tofu and vegetables is to think, "What would a carnivore do?" That's why we cut tofu into thick steaks and marinate it in a powerful miso sauce that doubles as a dressing for the finished product. This is tofu for vegetarians and meateaters alike.

- ¼ matcha powder
- ¼ cup white miso
- ¼ cup sugar
- 2 tbsp soy sauce
- 2 tbsp rice wine vinegar
- ¼ cup water
- 2 cloves garlic, minced
- 2 tbsp minced ginger
- 1 block firm tofu (12 oz), sliced into ¼"-thick steaks
- 1 head broccoli, florets broken into 1" pieces
- Oil for coating
- Salt and black pepper to taste
- Metal skewers, or wood skewers soaked in water for 30 minutes
- 4 cups cooked brown rice
- Toasted sesame seeds for garnish

→ Combine the m̶a̶r̶i̶n̶

̶s̶h̶a̶r̶p̶ ̶p̶o̶i̶n̶t̶ ̶t̶h̶r̶o̶u̶g̶h̶ each stalk to
hold it in place.

→ Remove the tofu from the bag, reserving the marinade.
Grill the tofu, turning once, for about 10 minutes, until caramelized and lightly crisp on the outside. Cook the broccoli, turning,
for about 12 minutes, until the florets are browned and
the stalks have softened.

→ Divide the rice among 4 bowls. Top with the tofu and broccoli,
then drizzle some of the leftover marinade over the top.
Garnish with sesame seeds.

MAKES 4 SERVINGS

390 calories / 10 g fat (2.5 g saturated) / 720 mg sodium

SNACKS

Artful 'Choke Dip

Green Superfoods

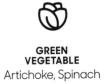

**GREEN
VEGETABLE**

Artichoke, Spinach

**GREEN
FRUIT**

Lemon

**GREEN
FAT**

Olive Oil

This classic dip is normally hijacked by a roguish team of full-fat mayo and cream cheese; somewhere, hidden within, lie token amounts of spinach and artichoke. Here, we turn that ratio on its head, plus use a flavorful olive oil–based mayo to cut calories and boost nutrition. Chiles bring some extra heat to the equation, while toasted wheat pitas work as super scoopers. Overall, this reimagined appetizer packs an amazing 14 grams of fiber.

4   large whole-wheat pitas

½   tbsp butter

1   onion, finely chopped

3   cloves garlic, finely chopped

1   jar (12 oz) artichoke hearts in water, drained and chopped

1   box (16 oz) chopped frozen spinach, thawed

1   can (4 oz) roasted green chiles, drained and chopped

2   Tbsp olive oil mayonnaise (made by both Kraft and Hellmann's)

2   tbsp whipped cream cheese

     Juice of 1 lemon

     Salt and black pepper to taste

→ Cut the pitas into 6 to 8 wedges e~~
  Spread on 2 bal~~

~~u wedges.

SERVINGS

270 calories / 10 g fat (2.5 g saturated) / 520 mg sodium

Greek Yogurt Green Tea Panna Cotta with Strawberry Quinoa Crumble

Green Superfoods

GREEN TEA

GREEN FRUIT
Strawberries

GREEN PROTEIN
Greek Yogurt

FOR THE PANNA COTTA:

- 1½   teaspoons unflavored gelatin
- 1   tablespoon water
- 1   cup whole milk
- ⅓   cup sugar
- 1   vanilla bean
- 1   teaspoon matcha green tea powder
- 1   cup buttermilk
- 1   cup 2% Greek yogurt

FOR THE QUINOA CRUMBLE:

- ½   cup rolled oats
- 2   tablespoons quinoa flakes

→ Combine milk and sugar in small saucepan; bring to a simmer. While milk heats, slit the vanilla bean lengthwise and scrape the insides into the milk mixture. (It'll look a little grainy, but don't worry. It will break up as you continue.) Add the matcha powder. Cook, stirring continuously, until the sugar is dissolved, about 1 minute. Remove from heat and stir in the gelatin until dissolved.

→ In a medium bowl, whisk the buttermilk with the yogurt, then add the warm milk and whisk until smooth. Pour the mixture into 4 8-oz cups (fill only halfway) and refrigerate for 3 hours, or until set.

→ While panna cotta is cooling, preheat oven to 350 degrees. Combine the oats, quinoa flakes, almond flour, sugar, and nutmeg in a food processor and pulse several times to combine. (Do not overmix.) Add the cold butter, and pulse until the butter is evenly combined and the mixture is crumbly.

→ Spread crumble mixture evenly on a parchment-lined baking sheet and bake for 10 minutes. Stir and bake for another 10 minutes, or until dark golden brown. Let cool completely.

→ Remove cooled panna cotta from refrigerator, cover with a layer of sliced strawberries, and top with crumble mixture.

MAKES 6 SERVINGS

253 calories / 10 g fat (5.4 g saturated) / 119 mg sodium / 24 g sugar

THE *17-DAY GREEN TEA DIET* RECIPES

Green Tea Yogurt
Green Superfoods

**GREEN
TEA**

**GREEN
FRUIT**
Strawberries

**GREEN
FAT**
Nuts

**GREEN
PROTEIN**
Greek Yogurt

1   8-ounce container organic 2% Greek yogurt

1   teaspoon matcha green tea powder

½   cup chopped strawberries

½   cup chopped nuts

1   tablespoon honey

➜ Place yogurt in a serving bowl. Using sifter, sift the matcha powder over the yogurt and whisk until evenly blended. Top with chopped strawberries and nuts. Drizzle with honey.

MAKES 2 SERVINGS

273 calories / 14 g fat (2.6 g saturated) / 38 mg sodium / 16 g sugar

FOR WEIGHT LOSS

Would you pay top dollar for a comedy performance by...Peele? Or expect a great film from a singular Coen brother? Or rock to the sounds of just one of those robots from Daft Punk?

There's a reason why people love the music of the Stones more than the work of Jagger or Richards alone: Amazing things happen when two great collaborators work in tandem to create magic. That's true in art, and it's just as true in nutrition. More and more research confirms what great chefs and home cooks have always known: Foods weren't meant to be eaten alone. They're meant to work in partnership, each bringing its own set of unique flavors (and nutrients) to create the perfect weight-loss meal.

Case in point: In early 2015, a study published in *The American Journal of Clinical Nutrition* reported that salads were more nutritionally potent if you added eggs to them. The reason: The eggs made it easier for your body to absorb carotenoids, the pigments that give veggies their color—and help you fight weight gain. Here are seven other ideal collaborators, each bringing its own unique nutritional talents to help keep you slim.

WEIGHT-LOSS COMBO 7
TUNA + GINGER

Want to look better on the beach? Look no further than the ocean—or at least the oceanside sushi joint. Pairing a tuna roll or a few pieces of tuna sashimi with ginger can help your belly look smaller immediately. The ginger accelerates gastric emptying, which helps diminish that "food baby" look rapidly, and it also blocks several genes and enzymes in the body that promote bloat-causing inflammation. Tuna's role here is critical, too: It's a primo source of docosahexaenoic acid, a type of omega-3 fat that can ward off stress chemicals that promote flab storage and downregulate fat genes in the stomach, stopping belly-fat cells from growing larger.

MAKE A POWER COMBO: Place the ginger atop your brown rice sushi—but lay off the soy sauce. A single tablespoon has more than 1,000 milligrams of belly-bloating sodium—more than a Big Mac!

WEIGHT-LOSS COMBO 6
SPINACH + AVOCADO OIL

If you're tiring of your usual go-to spinach-and-olive-oil salad, mix things up with avocado oil. Made from pressed—yes— avocados, it's rich in heart-healthy monounsaturated fats that may help improve cholesterol and ward off hunger. It also contains vitamins B and E and bloat-banishing potassium. Meanwhile, the high-volume, low-calorie spinach will fill you up without filling you out. And studies show that women who eat foods with high water content, such as leafy greens, have lower BMIs and smaller waistlines than those who don't. Go green to get lean.

COMBO

CORN + BEANS

While eating "a musical fruit" may not sound like the best way to lose weight or reduce bloat, hear us out. A calorie-restricted diet that includes four weekly servings of protein-and fiber-rich legumes has been proven to aid weight loss more effectively than a diet that doesn't include beans, according to Spanish researchers. And pairing beans with corn can help boost the slimming effect. Corn—like bananas and cold pasta—contains resistant starch, a carb that dodges digestion. In turn, the body isn't able to absorb as many of its calories or glucose, a nutrient that's stored as fat if it's not burned off. Music to our ears.

MAKE A POWER COMBO: Make a quick and easy corn and bean side dish. Combine salt- and BPA-free cans of corn and beans in a saucepan and warm over medium heat. Season with ground pepper and cilantro. Add the mixture to greens for a waist-trimming salad, use it as a flavorful topper for grilled chicken, or load the mixture into a toasted whole-grain pita pocket for a quick, on-the-go lunch.

WEIGHT-LOSS COMBO 4
HONEYDEW + RED GRAPES

Fight fat and banish bloating with a fruit salad composed of honey-dew and red grapes. Melon is a natural diuretic, so it helps fight the water retention responsible for making you look puffy even though you have a toned stomach. Red grapes add fuel to the better-belly fire because they contain an antioxidant called anthocyanin that helps calm the action of fat-storage genes. This dynamic duo makes for a delicious, healthy dessert, perfect for summer.

MAKE A POWER COMBO: Throw both into a fruit salad—and add some other green, red, orange, and yellow fruits.

WEIGHT-LOSS COMBO 3
CAYENNE + CHICKEN

You feel like chicken tonight? Good for you: Protein-rich foods like poultry not only boost satiety but also help people eat less at subsequent meals, according to research. And adding cayenne pepper fires up your fat burn. A compound in the pepper called capsaicin has proven to suppress appetite and boost the body's ability to convert food to energy. Daily consumption of capsaicin speeds up abdominal fat loss, a study published in *The American Journal of Clinical Nutrition* found.

MAKE A POWER COMBO: Just 1 gram of red pepper (about ½ teaspoon) can help manage appetite and increase calorie burn after a meal, according to a study at Purdue University. So go beyond chicken and season grilled fish, meats, and eggs with a pinch of red chili pepper.

WEIGHT

...... potatoes

......g than fiber-rich brown rice and oatmeal—and they're a good source of bloat-banishing potassium, so you'll look slimmer almost immediately. Just be sure to skip the butter in favor of pepper. Piperine, the powerful compound that gives black pepper its taste, may interfere with the formation of new fat cells—a reaction known as adipogenesis—which can help trim your waist, zap body fat, and lower cholesterol levels.

MAKE A POWER COMBO: Enjoy half a baked potato with a bit of olive oil and fresh pepper—and not just as a side dish. It can be a snack, too!

WEIGHT-LOSS COMBO 1
GREEN TEA + CINNAMON

Next time you're brewing up a cup, fight fat and ward off diet-derailing hunger by stirring your tea with a stick of cinnamon. Cinnamon is flavorful, practically calorie-free, and contains powerful antioxidants that are proven to reduce the accumulation of belly flab. Pair that with an appetite-suppressing cup of green tea, and you're losing weight first thing in the morning.

MAKE A POWER COMBO: If you're using loose-leaf tea, add crushed cinnamon sticks into the strainer for an even better taste and all the same weight-loss benefits.

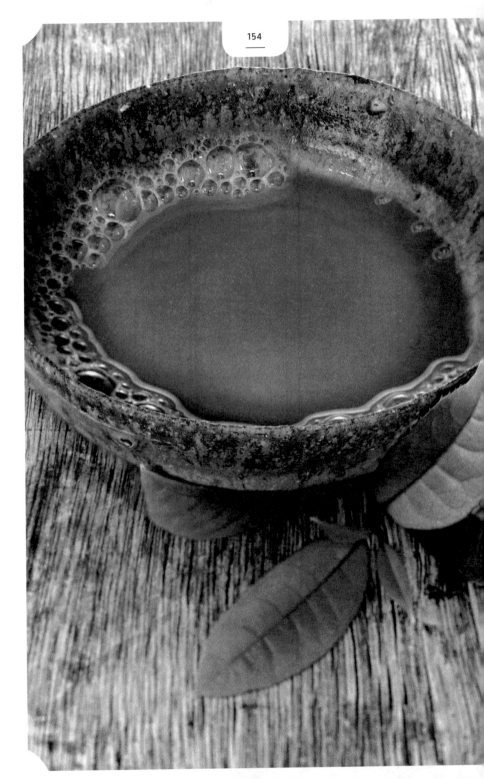

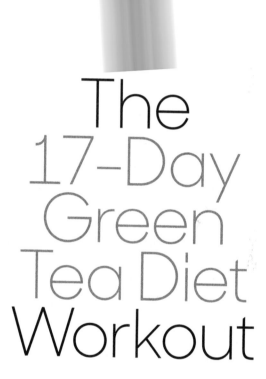

The 17-Day Green Tea Diet Workout

A simple slim-down fitness plan
that takes your weight loss
to the next level

THE *17-DAY GREEN TEA DIET* WORKOUT

t's easy to be intimidated by the hard-core fitness crowd that seems to hang around every gym, every running track, every spin class and yoga studio. Whereas a few years ago we all seemed to be feeling our way around fitness, nowadays the world seems divided into haves (abs) and have-nots.

And with so many options available—aqua aerobics to Zumba—it's hard to know what workout is right for you or whether you've found the right gym, the right equipment, or the right instructor.

But there's one piece of equipment that you definitely have at hand. In fact, your hands are actually attached to it right now. By using your own body weight, you can get a workout that's just as effective as anything designed for a high-priced gym. And since the best workout in the world is the one you'll actually do, it makes sense to follow a program that you can do anywhere—on the road, at home, visiting relatives, or while gorging on a 14-hour *House of Cards* binge fest.

These two workouts can be added into your weekly routine as time allows. For maximum impact, do Workout #1 three days a week, after your first cup of tea but before your first meal or smoothie of the day. This approach ensures that you'll be using stored fat, not your most recent snack, to fuel the workout. The entire workout takes just 10 minutes, including warm-up and cooldown.

Do Workout #2 on off days, or on days when your energy levels are simply flagging and a full workout just isn't in the cards. Because it takes only seven minutes, it can fit into even the most hectic of schedules.

THE 17-DAY GREEN TEA DIET

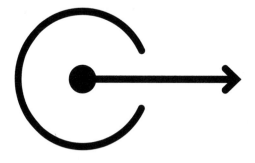

This workout is based upon the HIIT training protocol, which has been the subject of extensive research over the past few decades. HIIT stands for high-intensity interval training, and it involves short bursts of intense activity divided by rest periods half as long as the activity period. While traditional HIIT workouts are often performed on stationary bikes, this one involves body-weight exercises, thus maximizing aerobic efficiency while working the muscles of the entire body as well.

THE HIIT
BODY WEIGHT WORKOUT

Every exercise is to be performed as fast as possible without losing form.

3 MINUTES	Warm up on a stationary cardio machine, do jumping jacks, or jog in place
20 SECONDS	Run in Place (high knees)
10 SECONDS	Rest
20 SECONDS	Mountain Climbers
10 SECONDS	Rest
20 SECONDS	Skater Jumps (side-to-side, mimicking a skater's stride)
10 SECONDS	Rest
20 SECONDS	Push-ups (elbows close to sides of body)
10 SECONDS	Rest

Repeat work/rest cycle once

---

3 MINUTES	Cool down with any of above warm-up movements for 5 minutes

, without stopping for the duration of your warm-up.

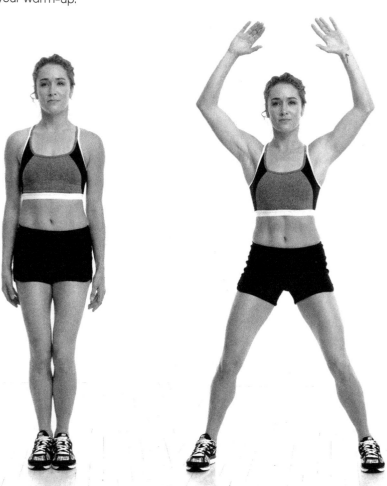

THE *17-DAY GREEN TEA DIET* WORKOUT

② RUN IN PLACE (HIGH KNEES)

Run in place, bringing your knees up as high as you can and pumping your legs as quickly as you can, for 20 seconds.

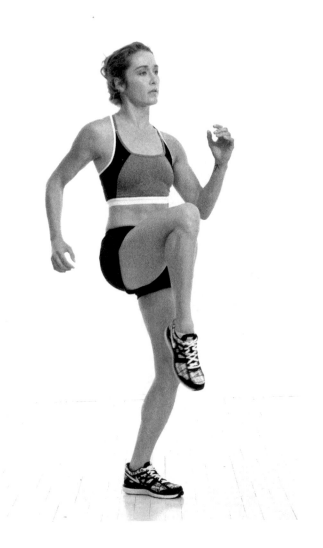

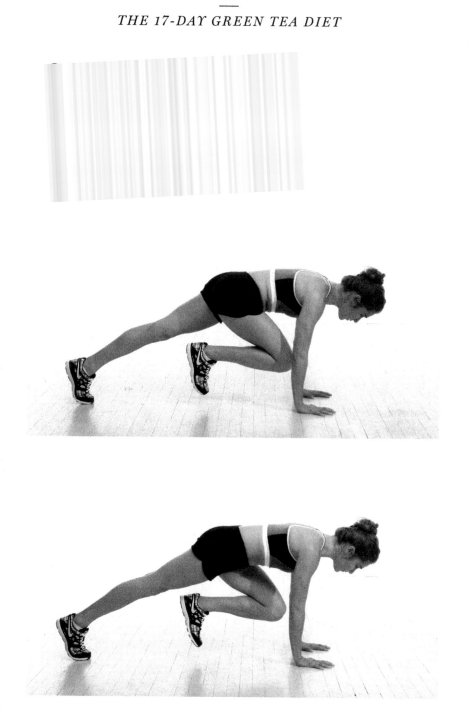

❹ SKATER JUMPS

From a crouched position with your feet close together, take a sideways leap to your left, landing on your left foot, with your right foot sweeping behind it, your left arm sweeping in front of your midsection, and your left arm sweeping out to the side. Now hop to your right, landing on your right foot and reversing the position of your other limbs. This should be a smooth, comfortable motion that mimics the movement of a speed skater in action.

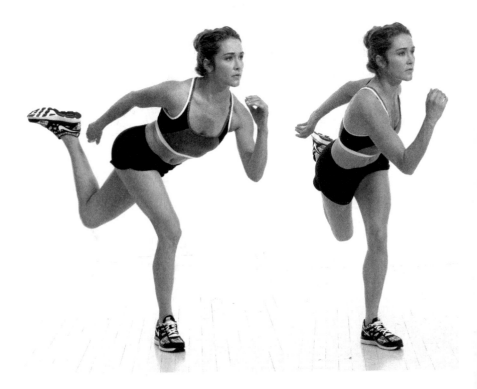

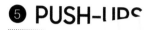

⑤ PUSH-UPS

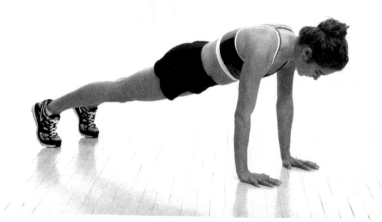

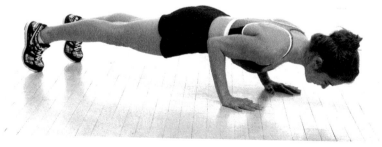

The Seven-Minute Ab Solution

Nobody loves working their abs, but adding an extra seven minutes onto your workout could make a huge difference in your core strength and definition. This workout is designed to get your abs to pop in just seven minutes a day. It's a great workout to do on days when you're not working out; make it your first-thing-in-the-morning thing, and you'll find your entire body getting stronger and more functional.

Use a timer and spend one minute performing each exercise. Do as many reps as you can in that time, resting as needed. Every time one minute is up, go on to the next exercise, no matter how little rest you've had. For the plank and side planks, hold the positions for one minute each, or as long as you can. Each time you repeat the workout, try to perform more reps for each exercise.

❶ PUSHUP WALK

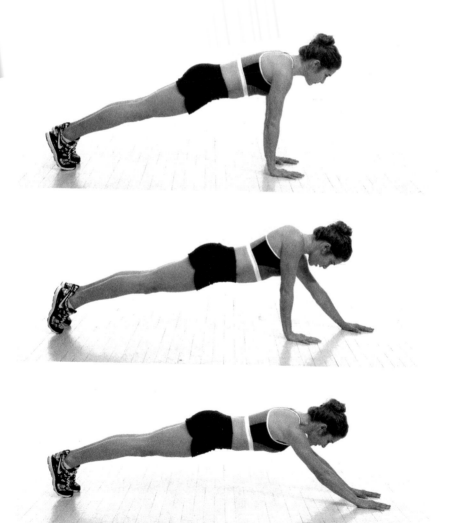

THE *17-DAY GREEN TEA DIET* WORKOUT

❷ LEG RAISE

Lie on the floor on your back and reach back to grab a chair, bench, or partner's legs for support. Keeping your legs straight, raise your legs up in the air until they're vertical. Lower them back down but stop an inch above the floor.

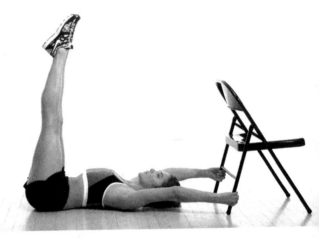

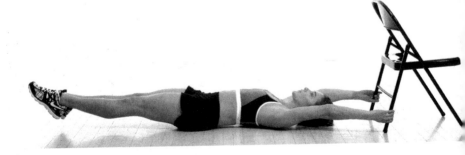

❸ REACHING CRU...

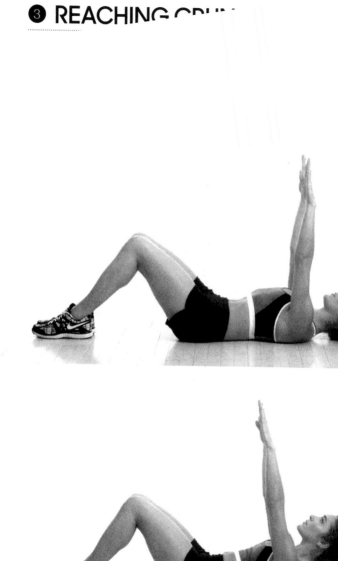

❹ FLUTTER KICK

Lie on the floor on your back with your legs straight and your arms by your sides. Contract your abs and raise your legs off the floor a few

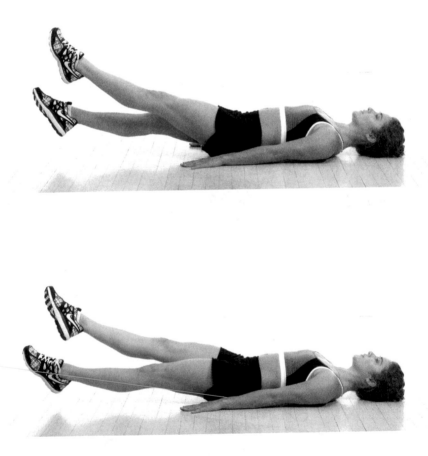

⑤ PLANK

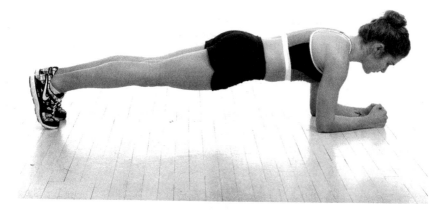

❻ SIDE PLANK (LEFT)

Lie on your left side, resting your left forearm on the floor for support. Raise your hips up so that your body forms a straight line and brace your abs—your weight should be on your left forearm and the edge of your left foot. Hold the position for as long as you can.

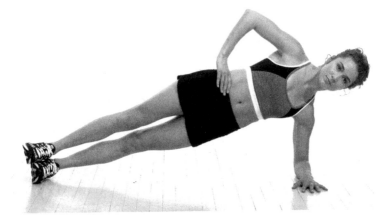

❼ SIDE PLANK (RIGHT)

Perform the side plank as described above but on your right side.

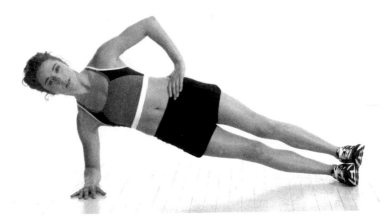

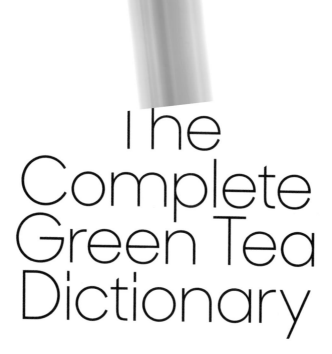

The Complete Green Tea Dictionary

Japanese Green Teas

GYOKURO Considered the finest of the Japanese green teas. Gyokuro leaves are flat and pointed, providing a smooth taste with a light fragrance. To ensure their mild taste, these leaves spend the last few weeks of their growth cycle in the shade, out of direct sunlight.

SENCHA The table wine of Japanese green tea, this is the most commonly used everyday variety. Quality can vary widely.

BANCHA Harvested very late in the season, bancha leaves are very large and sturdy. The stems and stalks are also included, so when it brews, bancha has a weaker flavor than most other, leaf-only teas.

MATCHA A bright-green powdered tea from the Uji region of Japan. It is higher in EGCG content than leaf tea, and used in the traditional Japanese tea ceremony. Less expensive versions from China are typically brown and more bitter.

HOUJICHA These green tea leaves are roasted, giving them a brown color and a nutty flavor. The roasting process also lowers the caffeine levels of the tea.

KUKICHA Connoisseurs liken the taste of kukicha to that of chestnuts. The unusual flavor comes from the fact that the twigs of the tea tree are included in the mix.

GENMAICHA Also known as "popcorn tea," genmaicha is a sencha tea that is pan-fired and then blended with toasted, hulled rice. The nickname "popcorn" comes from the fact that the rice often pops while it's being toasted. The combination gives this tea a comforting, nutty flavor, similar to oatmeal.

Chinese Green Teas

PU-ERH Also spelled Pu'er, this aged, dark tea from the Yunnan Province is unique in that the leaves are fermented after they are dried and rolled, then formed into bricks or cakes. Pu-erh may come in as many as ten or more grades, determined by leaf size and quantity, with the higher numbered grades indicating older, broken, or less tender leaves; many bricks are made from a blend of different grades in order to create the most balanced flavor.

GUNPOWDER Primarily grown in the Zhejian Province of

China, this popular tea looks like littl...

...ewnat rare, this ... as Pi Lo Chun. It's grown alongside stone fruit trees like peach, plum and apricot, which allows it to pick up the fragrance of the fruit.

SNOWY MOUNTAIN JIAN
Grown at high altitude in the Chinese province of Yunnan (hence the name), this tea is known for its long leaves and full-bodied flavor, which is closer to a black tea than a traditional green.

HYSON LUCKY DRAGON
Perhaps the most full-bodied of any green tea, Lucky Dragon can be recognized by its distinctive greenish-yellow color.

KAI HUA LONG DING
A high-quality tea from the Tiantai County region of China, it's known for its thick, short leaves and subtle flavor.

TIAN MU QING DING
The perfect tea for the forgetful, its fine, delicate leaves produce a sweet, light taste that is hard to over-steep.

XIN YANG MAO JIAN
Also known as "green tip," this tea from the Henan Province is brewed from very fine, delicate leaves.

MONKEY TEA
From the Anhui Province, monkey tea, also called Hou Kui, is grown amongst orchid plants, allowing its leaves to absorb the rich fragrance and flavor of the orchid flower.

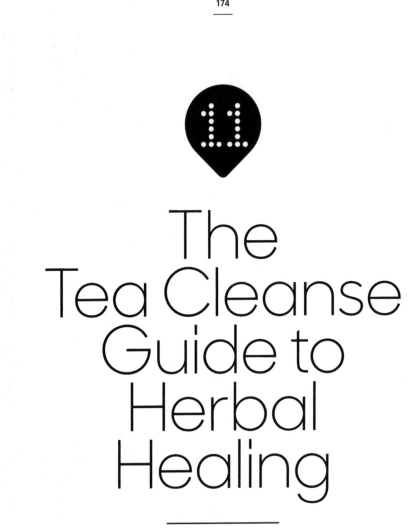

The Tea Cleanse Guide to Herbal Healing

There's a drug-free remedy for what ails you, from arthritis to headaches to the common cold.

..., espe-

... drugs.

Americans spend more per capita on medicines than any other developed country, and buy more generics, too—and even the generics can cost $80 and up, since prices rise and average of 5% a year. As a result, the natural-foods aisle is suddenly flooded with people trying to tell their cramp root from their dong quai. Vulnerable, hurting for money, we want to believe these cheaper remedies work. And do they?

This chapter tells you, definitively, which ones do—and which ones don't. We've combed through the most up-to-date research on botanical medicines, studying the latest breakthroughs and debunking the false claims. And we're happy to report that relief is here for cancer, diabetes, even jet lag.

The idea behind herbal remedies is wonderfully simple: Herbalists believe whole plants are more effective than the isolated elements and synthetic ingredients used in drugs—with the added bonus of fewer unintentional effects. Herbal medicines should be seriously considered for ailments like colds and flu, insomnia, autoimmune diseases—the worries that typically cause conventional docs to throw up their hands. Yet herbs are also proven to help ease the symptoms of more serious ailments, like heart disease and cancer.

Chinese, Egyptian, Indian, and indigenous American civilizations might say, "Welcome to the club, America, what took you so long?" If trends here continue, it won't be long before this "boom" becomes common practice. While still not fully accepted by Western medicine or every M.D., herbal medicine is now taught more in medical and pharmacy schools. Extensive studies are ongoing not just overseas but now in the United States. And because some medical doctors realize that plants are the source of many synthetic drugs, an increasing number accept that herbs have benefit.

Just how much benefit? In this chapter, we recommend only products that fared well in evidence-based or double-blind studies—giving an honest look at what to buy and what to avoid. This A-to-Z guide to herbal healing includes plants that can boost your mood, your energy, and your sex drive. As a sales pitch, it's irresistible; as medicine, it's sound.

What to Know Before You Buy

So, how safe are these products? And do they do what they promise? Well... it's tricky. Manufacturers do not need FDA approval to put their products on the market, and are allowed to put claims on the label, as long as they also note that the FDA hasn't approved the claim.

Once a product is on the market, the FDA does monitor its quality and safety, and if it's deemed unsafe, it can issue a warning or require the maker or distributor to remove the product from the marketplace. (In Europe and Australia, herbal products must provide scientific proof before any medicinal claims can be printed on labels.)

These guidelines do not, however, guarantee that an herb is safe for anyone to take—there may be dangerous interactions with other herbs or drugs, so always tell your medical doctor, and the herbal dispensary, about any drugs or herbal supplements you're on. Also:

Do your own research

...ger. Also be careful if you ... ... immunosuppressant drugs—drugs that are used to suppress the immune system after a transplant or to control symptoms of autoimmune disease such as lupus and type-1 diabetes—such as corticosteroids (prednisone). Herbs that boost immunity, such as licorice, astragalus, and ginseng, may counteract these drugs.

Look for reputable brands.

Many good companies are represented in these pages; try to buy from companies that have been in business for a long time and have an established reputation.

Learn how to read labels.

A reputable brand will not just tell you its product will cure your headache—it should also tell you how, and you should be able to find ingredient descriptions and actions on the product website. Then you can cross-reference with unbiased, evidence-based research.

Follow label instructions.

Duh. Don't think that if a little works well, a lot will work better. Just don't do it. And don't mix one herb with another herb, unless a professional tells you to.

Be smart.

If you're pregnant or nursing, or have severe allergies or ailments, then don't take herbs without talking to your doctor. Don't give to children without talking to your doctor.

Tell your medical doctor what you're up to.

Unfortunately, a *New England Journal of Medicine* study found that 70% of people (mostly well-educated and with a high income) do not tell their doctors that they are using complementary or alternative treatments.

Healing Herbs
A-to-Z

This is it: The List. The 23 herbs that have been proven to work—with a few bliss boosters and serenity savers as a bonus. Stick to the dosages specified here, in the studies, or on the label—and make sure to tell your doctor about any herbs you plan to take, especially if you are pregnant or nursing, have a chronic condition, or take medication regularly; remember that even though herbs are natural, they can still be contraindicated.

1 ALOE VERA *(Aloe barbadensis)*

BEST FOR → Burns

Aloe vera is the herb for minor (second-degree) burns, confirmed by a 2009 *Surgery Today* study, among others that have shown aloe vera gel has a dramatic effect on burns, wounds and other skin conditions. The gel provides a protective layer for the affected area, and speeds healing due to aloecin B, which stimulates the immune system. The gel also can be used orally for ulcers and irritable bowel syndrome and as a laxative; it creates an internal protective coating and also stimulates the digestion.

DOSAGE: Apply 100% pure gel to burns several times a day—or, better yet, keep a potted plant on your ~~~ ~· ·

BOSWELLIA *(Boswellia serrata)*

BEST FOR → **Arthritis and joint injuries**

Also known as Indian frankincense, this gummy resin has been clinically proven to have strong anti-inflammatory effects. Boswellia is known to reduce congestion and heat (kapha and pitta elements in ayurveda) in the joints, and is also used to promote appetite and digestion.

In a 2008 study published in *Arthritis Research & Therapy*, researchers gave people with osteoarthritis of the knee an extract of boswellia (5-Loxin). After three months, the herb group showed significantly greater relief than a group given a placebo.

DOSAGE: Take one 300-milligram capsule three times a day, with food.

3 ECHINACEA *(Echinacea angustifolia)*

BEST FOR → **Common cold**

Studies on the effectiveness of echinacea for treating the common cold have been mixed. The largest so far was in 2012 at Cardiff University Common Cold Centre in the U.K., which found that three doses daily, taken for four months reduced the number of colds, and reduced the duration by 26%. The study was peer-reviewed and published in the journal *Evidence-Based Complementary and Alternative Medicine*. The study was funded by the Swiss manufacturers of Echinaforce. But many experts advise ignoring the naysayers, and following traditional usage.

"Native Americans used *Echinacea angustifolia*—not *Echinacea purpurea*—and they used only the root," explains Sheila Kingsbury, N.D., chair of the Department of Botanical Medicine at Bastyr University in Seattle. "Clinically speaking, accessing the root is the best place to start. It can shorten the length of a cold significantly."

DOSAGE: One teaspoon of echinacea root glycerite liquid every two hours beginning at onset of symptoms; decrease the dose to once every three to four hours after symptoms ease.

4 EVENING PRIMROSE OIL *(Oenothera)*

BEST FOR → Eczema

Evening primrose seeds contain an oil with a high concentration of compounds rarely found in plants: the essential fatty acid gamma linolenic acid. There are more than 30 human studies reporting its benefits; in one, 1,207 patients found that the oil helped relieve the itching, swelling, crusting, and redness of eczema, which a 2013 University of Maryland Medical Center review confirms. It also has been found to lower blood pressure and reduce PMS and some multiple sclerosis symptoms when taken internally.

DOSAGE: Apply topically for skin conditions; follow label instructions for internal use.

5 FENNEL *(Foeniculum vulgare)*

BEST FOR → Intestinal gas

Fennel seeds contain phytonutrients that are thought to reduce spasms in small muscle fibers like those found in the intestines, helping to reduce gassiness. The aromatic quality of the seeds will also help freshen your breath. And a 2011 review published in *Pediatrics*, for instance, found that fennel tea can be useful for treating a baby's gas-caused colic.

DOSAGE: Chew a pinch of whole fennel seeds after a meal. Your body will let you know—with one last burst of gas—when to stop.

... cholesterol levels than men from age 45 on, according to the AHA. Flaxseed, which is rich in the omega-3 fat alpha-linoleic acid, may help lower it.

An Italian study of 40 male and female patients with cholesterol levels greater than 240 milligrams per deciliter found that consuming ground flaxseed (20 grams, or about 0.7 ounces, daily) could significantly lower levels of total and LDL cholesterol (the artery-clogging kind), while also improving the ratio of total cholesterol to HDL. (Low levels of HDL may be a greater risk factor for women, according to the AHA.) In a Harvard study of 76,763 women participating in the Nurses' Health Study, researchers also noted that women consuming a diet rich in alpha-linolenic acid seem to have a lower risk of dying from heart disease and stroke, compared with women whose diets were lacking this fat. Flaxseed also provides fiber; two tablespoons of ground flaxseed have 4 grams of fiber—almost 20% of the 25 grams recommended by the U.S. Department of Agriculture. Lignans, which are a particular type of fiber found in flaxseed, may also be beneficial for preventing breast and prostate cancer, according to preliminary studies. (Lignans are not present in flaxseed oil, however, notes integrative physician and herbalist Tieraona Low Dog, M.D.)

DOSAGE: Low Dog recommends adding 1 to 5 tablespoons of ground flaxseed to your diet several days a week; sprinkle it on cereal or yogurt, or stir it into protein shakes. Flaxseed oil—which must be kept refrigerated to prevent rancidity—should be added to salads and not used for cooking.

PRECAUTIONS: Flaxseed and its oil are safe if consumed in normal amounts, although they can produce a laxative effect. "If you eat huge amounts of flaxseed meal, you could develop cyanide toxicity, but this hasn't, to my knowledge, ever occurred in humans," says Low Dog.

7 GARLIC *(Allium sativum L.)*

BEST FOR → Ear infections and cancer prevention

Garlic's antibiotic compound, alliin, has no medicinal value until the herb is chewed, chopped or crushed. Then an enzyme transforms alliin into a powerful antibiotic called allicin. Raw garlic has the most antibiotic potency, but garlic still has benefits when cooked. Garlic is antimicrobial and anti-inflammatory, so it will treat any infection, but when combined with mullein oil (*Verbascum densiflorum*), it's especially effective for ear infections, says a 2010 report in *Natural News*. The mullein oil is soothing, and helps draw out fluid to relieve pain and decrease pressure. According to the National Cancer Institute, preliminary studies in 2008 suggest that garlic consumption may also reduce the risk of developing several types of cancer, especially those of the gastrointestinal tract.

DOSAGE: Put three drops of oil in each affected ear, two to three times a day as needed. (The oils are sold in a premixed formula.) For internal use, fresh garlic or capsules may be used; follow label directions.

PRECAUTIONS: Don't put drops—or anything else—into your ear if you think the eardrum may be perforated.

8 GINGER *(Zingiber officinale)*

BEST FOR: Nausea and vomiting

A Danish study showed that new sailors prone to motion sickness had less vomiting than a placebo group. Research published in *Obstetrics & Gynecology* found that 88% of nausea-plagued pregnant women got relief when they took 1 gram a day of ginger powder for no longer than four

...linked to normal ginger consumption, but powdered ginger may produce bloating or indigestion. Ginger may also exacerbate heartburn in pregnant women.

9 GINKGO *(Ginkgo biloba)*

BEST FOR: Alzheimer's and antidepressant-induced sexual problems

In a landmark study published in *The Journal of the American Medical Association*, researchers gave 202 people with Alzheimer's either a placebo or 120 milligrams a day of ginkgo extract. A year later, the ginkgo group retained more mental function. According to new research in rats (2013), supplementation with an extract from *Ginkgo biloba* may help to battle memory loss and cognitive impairments associated with dementia by encouraging the growth and development of neural stem cells. From upstairs to downstairs: In a University of California, San Francisco study, investigators gave 209 milligrams of ginkgo a day to 63 people suffering from antidepressant-induced sexual problems, including erection impairment, vaginal dryness and inability to reach orgasm; the herb helped 91% of the women and 76% of the men to return to normal sexual function.

DOSAGE: Traditional usage is 80 to 240 milligrams of a 50:1 standardized leaf extract daily or 30 to 40 milligrams of extract in a tea bag, prepared as a tea, for at least four to six weeks.

10 GINSENG

BEST FOR: Immune enhancement and diabetes

Many studies show that ginseng has "adaptogenic" powers, which means it helps the body adapt to stress and revs up the immune system. Most studies have used Panax *ginseng* (Asian ginseng). A 2013 University of Maryland review found that Asian ginseng may help boost the immune system, reduce risk of cancer and improve mental performance and wellbeing. And subjects who took daily doses of ginseng got fewer colds and less severe symptoms than a placebo group. Ginseng also reduces blood-sugar levels. A study in Toronto, Canada, found that Korean red ginseng improved glucose and insulin regulation in well-controlled type 2 diabetes. (Of course, diabetes requires professional treatment, so consult your physician about using ginseng.) Studies also have found ginseng supports liver function and one preliminary study suggests that American ginseng (*Panax quinquefolius*), in combination with ginkgo (*Ginkgo biloba*), may help treat ADHD.

DOSAGE: 500 milligrams daily, best for short-term, stressful events

PRECAUTIONS: Should not be taken for more than six weeks. Avoid caffeine when taking ginseng, and do not take if pregnant.

11 GOLDENROD (*Solidago virgaurea*)

BEST FOR: Nasal congestion

Goldenrod is particularly effective for treating congestion caused by allergies. Surprised? That's because goldenrod gets a bad rap. "People blame goldenrod for their allergies because they look across the field and see the beautiful yellow flowers," says herbalist Margi Flint, author of *The Practicing Herbalist*. "But it's the blooming ragweed they can't see that causes all the trouble. In nature, the remedy often grows right next to the cause." Also used for urinary infections and

THE 17-DAY GREEN TEA DIET

cystitis, and to flush out kid

..., an herbal antibiotic, is often marketed in combination with echinacea as a treatment for infections, but it is effective only in the digestive tract, not for colds or flu. A 2012 University of Maryland study reported in *Clinical Advisor* found that goldenseal is an effective antibacterial agent and an aid to digestion. For gastrointestinal infections (e.g., ulcers, food poisoning, infectious diarrhea), ask your doctor about using goldenseal in addition to medical therapies. Also can be used topically for wounds and infections.

DOSAGE: For internal use, take a 300-milligram capsule three times a day; apply a dilution as needed for external use.

PRECAUTIONS: Can be toxic if taken to excess. May interact with antidepressants and codeine. Do not use if pregnant, nursing or suffering from high blood pressure.

13 LAVENDER *(Lavandula angustifolia)*

BEST FOR: Headaches

"The scent of lavender triggers a calming response, releasing tension in the scalp muscles a bit, which eases the pain," explains Kingsbury Herbalist Rosemary Gladstar. She recommends using lavender oil in a pain-relieving foot soak: Add a few drops to a hot footbath, and then put a cold lavender-infused pack on the forehead. "This draws heat away from the head, and is guaranteed to make you feel better," she says.

DOSAGE: Dab a few drops of essential oil on each temple and rub some around the hairline. Breathe deeply and relax; repeat as needed.

PRECAUTIONS: Do not take the essential oil internally unless under the care of a professional.

14 LEMON BALM *(Melissa officinalis)*

BEST FOR: Anxiety and herpes

Science has shown that lemon balm is tranquilizing. Several double-blind studies have found that a 600-milligram dose promoted calm and reduced anxiety. The herb and its oil have been used in Alzheimer's special care units to calm those who are agitated. To decompress after a tough day, try a cup of lemon balm tea; for extra benefit, mix with chamomile.

Lemon balm also has antiviral properties and has been shown to reduce the healing time of both oral and genital herpes. German researchers gave people in the early stages of herpes simplex virus outbreaks lemon balm cream or a placebo. The herb group had milder outbreaks that healed faster.

DOSAGE: Available in capsule form, tincture, and essential oil; follow label instructions.

PRECAUTIONS: Do not take the essential oil internally unless under the care of a professional.

15 MEADOWSWEET *(Filipendula ulmaria)*

BEST FOR: Heartburn

The Native American herb, high in salicylic acid, calms inflammation in the stomach, often working within a day or two, says Sheila Kingsbury. "For people on protein pump inhibitors who are desperate to get their heartburn under control without medication, I have them drink one cup of meadowsweet tea a day, and that's all they need," she says. "They're always shocked that it's so easy."

DOSAGE: D

BEST FOR: Liver health

Silymarin in milk thistle seeds has a remarkable ability to protect the liver. This herb has been shown to help treat hepatitis and alcoholic cirrhosis. "In our analysis," says Mark Blumenthal, executive director of the American Botanical Council, "a clear majority of studies support milk thistle seed extract for liver conditions." A 2010 NIH-NC-CAM study on the effects of silymarin on hepatitis C hepatology showed multiple positive effects demonstrating its antiviral and anti-inflammatory properties. Because most drugs are metabolized through the liver, many herbalists recommend silymarin for anyone who takes liver-taxing medication.

DOSAGE: 500 milligrams daily for liver health; also can be steeped in a tea.

17 PSYLLIUM *(Plantago spp.)*

BEST FOR: Digestive problems

Psyllium is a tiny seed that contains mucilage, a soluble fiber that swells on exposure to water. For diarrhea, psyllium can absorb excess fluid in the gut. For constipation, psyllium adds bulk to stool, which presses on the colon wall and triggers the nerves that produce the urge to go. Also helps relieve hemorrhoids and helps remove toxins. May be used topically to draw out infections such as boils.

DOSAGE: Follow label directions; also available in capsule form.

PRECAUTIONS: When using psyllium, drink plenty of water; do not

THE GUIDE TO HERBAL HEALING

exceed recommended dose.

18 ST. JOHN'S WORT *(Hypericum perforatum)*

BEST FOR: Depression and pain

"Long before it was ever used for depression or anxiety, St. John's wort was used as a pain reliever and an anti-inflammatory for muscle pains, burns, and bruises," explains Rosemary Gladstar, adding that blending the oil with the alcohol-based tincture helps draw the active constituents into the skin for faster healing. For mild depression, St. John's wort often works as well as some antidepressants but with fewer swide effects. "We recently concluded a comprehensive review of the scientific literature on St. John's wort, and 21 of 23 studies support it for mild to moderate depression," says Blumenthal. It's not clear if St. John's wort is as effective as selective serotonin reuptake inhibitors (SSRIs) such as Prozac or Zoloft, but a 2013 Mayo Clinic overview states that scientific evidence supports its use for mild to moderate depression; for severe depression, the evidence remains unclear.

DOSAGE: For depression, studies showing benefits have used 600 to 1,800 milligrams a day; most have used 900 milligrams a day. For pain, make a liniment by mixing equal parts St. John's wort tincture and St. John's wort oil. (Most concoctions come in 2-ounce bottles.) Mix vigorously before using, apply topically to affected area (avoiding the eyes), and massage into skin as needed.

PRECAUTIONS: Stomach upset is possible, and St. John's wort interacts with many drugs, including possibly reducing the effectiveness of birth control pills; so seek professional advice if you are taking a prescription medication. Depression requires professional care; ask your physician about St. John's wort. May cause sensitivity to light.

placebo, a 25% tea tree oil solution or a 50% tea tree oil solution for four weeks. Results showed that the tea tree oil solutions were more effective than placebo. (In the 50% tea tree oil group, 64% were cured; in the 25% tea tree oil group, 55% were cured; in the placebo group, 31% were cured.) Also helpful for a range of vaginal yeast infections.

DOSAGE: Apply essential oil mixed with a base cream or carrier oil to skin; for vaginal infections, use suppositories.

PRECAUTIONS: Do not take the essential oil internally unless advised by a professional.

20 TRIPHALA *(Emblica officinalis, Terminalia chebula and Terminalia belerica)*

BEST FOR: Constipation and digestive problems

Triphala ("three fruits" in Sanskrit), a bowel-regulating formula in ayurvedic medicine, is a combination of the powdered fruits of amalaki, bibhitaki, and haritaki, all of which are rich sources of antioxidants with anti-inflammatory, adaptogenic, antistress, antibacterial, analgesic, anticancer and immune-enhancing properties. A 2012 review published in the *Chinese Journal of Integrative Traditional and Western Medicine* confirms the extensive healing properties of this amazing herbal compound.

"Triphala treats the entire digestive system, helping with constipation, hemorrhoids, diarrhea, indigestion, bloating and liver detoxification," explains ayurvedic herbalist Will Foster, L.Ac., who trained with traditional ayurvedic healers in India. Because it operates as a bowel tonic (helping to maintain proper function) rather than a laxative, triphala is safe to take every day.

DOSAGE: Take two to four 500-milligram tablets just before bedtime.

PRECAUTIONS: Do not take during pregnancy or if underweight; can cause weight loss.

21 TURMERIC *(Curcuma longa)*

BEST FOR: Arthritis and cancer prevention

Curcumin, the active compound that gives the spice turmeric its bright-gold color, has long been known as an anti-inflammatory and antioxidant. In combination with boswellia, ashwagandha and ginger, it may treat osteoarthritis, according to a study published in the *Journal of Clinical Rheumatology*. And a recent study published in the journal *Phytotherapy* Research found curcumin to be "comparable" in efficacy to diclofenac sodium, a prescription anti-inflammatory, for treating rheumatoid arthritis.

The American Cancer Society has reported that large studies are being conducted to see how curcumin might prevent and treat cancer; one of the challenges is that it doesn't absorb well from the intestines, but that could be an advantage for targeting cancer precursors in the colon and rectum. For women with recurrent breast cancer, curcumin might prove especially useful; animal models have shown that curcumin may help prevent metastasis, even after failed treatment with the drug tamoxifen. In women with HER2-positive cancer, curcuminoids also seemed to behave much like the highly successful chemotherapy drug Herceptin, although research is very preliminary.

DOSAGE: It's best to get your curcumin by using turmeric in curries and other foods. If you aren't a fan of Indian food, take one 500-milligram capsule of curcumin—standardized to 95% curcuminoids—each day.

PRECAUTIONS: Side effects are rare but include flatulence, diarrhea and heartburn. Do not take turmeric if you're on blood thinners.

good clinical studies on the use of umckaloabo for treating bronchitis as well as tonsillitis," he says, adding that taking umckaloabo at the onset of symptoms will bring relief within a day or two. Recent German studies of the preparation found that it significantly reduced symptoms and duration of colds and cough.

DOSAGE: Take as drops, syrups, chewable tablets or sprays. Follow package instructions.

23 WHITE WILLOW BARK *(Salix alba)*

BEST FOR: Pain relief

White willow bark contains salicin, a close chemical relative of aspirin. A study in *Phytomedicine* followed people with severe back pain for 18 months. In the group taking white willow bark, 40% were pain-free after just four weeks; the same was true of only 18% of the second group, who were allowed to take whatever prescription drugs they wanted. In another well-designed study of nearly 200 people with low back pain, those who received willow bark experienced a significant improvement in pain compared to those who received placebo. People who received higher doses of willow bark (240 milligrams salicin) had more significant pain relief than those who received low doses (120 milligrams salicin). It has also been shown to relieve arthritis, inflammation, headaches and fever and hot flashes.

DOSAGE: Follow label directions; the bark can be made into a tea.

PRECAUTIONS: Like aspirin, willow bark can cause stomach distress, and shouldn't be given to children or used if pregnant or breast-feeding. Avoid if you are allergic to aspirin.

NOW READ THIS!

Discover all the great books from Eat This, Not That! and David Zinczenko, plus ebooks, apps and more.

No matter who you are (or what you love to eat!), we have a fast-and-easy plan that will help you lose weight and look and feel better than ever, all without sacrificing your favorite foods.

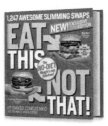

Eat This, Not That! Arm yourself with our annual guides to life-changing food swaps.

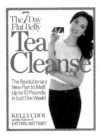

The 7-Day Flat-Belly Tea Cleanse Boost your metabolism, melt belly fat, and reduce stress in just one week!

The 17-Day Green Tea Diet The easiest, least expensive, most effective weight-loss plan on the planet

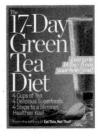

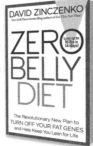

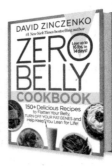

Zero Belly Diet The revolutionary new plan to turn off your fat genes and keep you lean for life

Zero Belly Cookbook 150+ delicious recipes to flatten your belly fast

www.ShopEatThisNotThat.com